NOTES ON CARDIORESPIRATORY DISEASES OF THE DOG AND CAT

NOTES ON CARDIORESPIRATORY DISEASES OF THE DOG AND CAT

Second Edition

Mike Martin MVB DVC MRCVS

RCVS Specialist in Veterinary Cardiology
Veterinary Cardiorespiratory Centre
Thera House
Kenilworth
Warwickshire
www.martinreferrals.com

Dr Brendan M Corcoran MVB DipPharm PhD MRCVS

Senior Lecturer
Director of the Hospital for Small Animals
Easter Bush Veterinary Centre
Royal (Dick) School of Veterinary Studies
University of Edinburgh
Roslin
Scotland

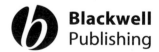
Blackwell Publishing

© 2006 Mike Martin and Brendan Corcoran

Editorial Offices:
Blackwell Publishing Ltd, 9600 Garsington Road, Oxford OX4 2DQ, UK
   Tel: +44 (0)1865 776868
Blackwell Publishing Professional, 2121 State Avenue, Ames, Iowa 50014-8300, USA
   Tel: +1 515 292 0140
Blackwell Publishing Asia, 550 Swanston Street, Carlton, Victoria 3053, Australia
   Tel: +61 (0)3 8359 1011

First published as Cardiorespiratory Diseases of the Dog and Cat in 1997 by Blackwell Science Ltd

ISBN-10: 1-4051-2264-1
ISBN-13: 978-1-4051-2264-1

Library of Congress Cataloging-in-Publication Data

Martin, Mike W. S.
   Notes on cardiorespiratory diseases of the dog and cat / Mike Martin, Brendan M. Corcoran.–
2nd ed.
      p. cm.
   Rev. ed. of: Cardiorespiratory diseases of the dog and cat. 1996.
   Includes bibliographical references and index.
   ISBN-13: 978-1-4051-2264-1 (alk. paper)
   ISBN-10: 1-4051-2264-1 (alk. paper)
   1. Dogs–Diseases.   2. Cats–Diseases.   3. Cardiopulmonary system–Diseases.   I. Corcoran,
Brendan M.   II. Martin, Mike W. S. Cardiorespiratory diseases of the dog and cat.   III. Title.

   SF992.C37M375 2005
   636.7'08961–dc22

                                                                            2005014103

A catalogue record for this title is available from the British Library

Set in 9/11.5pt Sabon
by Graphicraft Limited, Hong Kong
Printed and bound in India
by Replika Press Pvt Ltd.

The publisher's policy is to use permanent paper from mills that operate a sustainable forestry
policy, and which has been manufactured from pulp processed using acid-free and elementary
chlorine-free practices. Furthermore, the publisher ensures that the text paper and cover board
used have met acceptable environmental accreditation standards.

For further information on Blackwell Publishing, visit our website:
www.BlackwellVet.com

CONTENTS

Summary of Cardiopulmonary Resuscitation – inside back cover

PREFACE

In coming to terms with the challenge of updating this book, it has been striking how out-dated the first edition (1997) had become. This second edition has allowed us to significantly update the facts in many areas, particularly in relation to cardiology. Such rapid developments in veterinary medicine make it very difficult for the practitioner to keep up to date. This book is primarily intended for use by the practitioner and under-graduates, and hopefully we have made it concise and easy to read.

We have included many points, tips and ideas that we think will be of use to the prac-tising veterinarian, and have based this on our personal experience. Our ideas about the diagnosis and treatment of cardiorespiratory diseases have developed and evolved over many years, and we hope our practical experience is evident throughout the text. We have concentrated on the common diseases and omitted many of the rarer conditions.

We do hope you find this book useful. If you do, please tell your colleagues, if not please tell us.

Mike Martin and
Brendan Corcoran 2005

ACKNOWLEDGEMENTS AND DEDICATION

We would like to thank our colleagues, practitioners and our peers, who have undoubtedly influenced our gathering of knowledge and experience that is laid down in this text.

We would also like to thank Blackwell Science for their patience – we evidently didn't realise how much updating this book required and how long it was going to take.

We would like to dedicate this book to our families:

Mary, David, Dennis and Sean (MWSM)
Mary, Paul and Éoin (BC)

ABBREVIATIONS

2-D	two-dimensional
Aa	alveolar-arterial (gradient)
Ao	aorta
ACE	angiotensin converting enzyme
ACTH	adrenocorticotrophic hormone
ACP	acepromazine
AF	atrial fibrillation
AKA	also known as
ASD	atrial septal defect
AS	aortic stenosis
AV	atrioventricular
BAL	bronchoalveolar lavage
bid	twice daily
Ca^{++}	calcium
CAV-2	canine adenovirus-2
CB	chronic bronchitis
CHF	congestive heart failure
Cl$^-$	chloride
CP	*Chlamydophila psittaci*
CPA	cardiopulmonary arrest
CPR	cardiopulmonary resuscitation
CRI	constant rate infusion
CTS	chronic tracheobronchial syndrome
DC	direct current
DCM	dilated cardiomyopathy
DIC	disseminated intravascular coagulation
DV	dorsoventral
ECG	electrocardiograph
ELISA	enzyme-linked immunosorbent assay
EPSS	E-point to septal separation
ET	ejection time
FB	foreign body
FCV	feline calici virus
FeLV	feline leukaemia virus
FIV	feline immunodeficiency virus
FIP	feline infectious peritonitis
FRV	feline rhinotracheitis virus
FS	fractional shortening
GA	general anaesthesia
GSD	German Shepherd
HCM	hypertrophic cardiomyopathy
HOCM	hypertrophic obstructive cardiomyopathy
i/m	intramuscular
Iu	international unit
i/v	intravenous
IVSd	interventricular septal diameter in diastole
IVSs	interventricular septal diameter in systole
J	joule
K$^+$	potassium
kg	kilogram

kV	kilovolt
L1 to L5	stage 1 to 5 larvae
LA	left atrium
LBB	left bundle branch
LV	left ventricle
LVd	left ventricular internal diameter in diastole
LVs	left ventricular internal diameter in systole
LVOT	left ventricular outflow tract
LVPwd	left ventricular posterior wall thickness in diastole
LVPws	left ventricular posterior wall thickness in systole
mA	milliamp
mAs	milliampsecond
MEA	mean electrical axis
MEq	milliequivalent
mg	milligram
MIMI	microscopic intramural myocardial infarction
ml	millilitre
mmol	millimole
MR	mitral regurgitation
Na^+	sodium
ng	nanogram
$PaO_2/PaCO_2$	arterial partial pressure of oxygen/carbon dioxide
PCV	packed cell volume
PDA	patent ductus arteriosus
PEP	pre-ejection pause
per os	orally
PIE	pulmonary infiltrate with eosinophils
PMI	point of maximum intensity
PS	pulmonic stenosis
q	every
qid	four times daily
RA	right atrium
RBB	right bundle branch
RCM	restrictive cardiomyopathy
RV	right ventricle
SA	sinoatrial
SAM	systolic anterior motion
SAS	subaortic stenosis
S/C	sub-cutaneous
sid	once daily
SG	specific gravity
SPO_2	percent oxygenation saturation by pulse oximetry
SVPC	supraventricular premature complex
SVT	supraventricular tachycardia
T4	thyroxine
TG	triglyceride
tid	three times daily
TR	tricuspid regurgitation
TSH	thyroid stimulating hormone
μg	microgram
URTI	upper respiratory tract infection
VD	ventrodorsal
VF	ventricular fibrillation
VPC	ventricular premature complex
VSD	ventricular septal defect
VT	ventricular tachycardia
WHW	West Highland White (Terrier)
WPW	Wolff-Parkinson-White (syndrome)

SECTION 1
INVESTIGATION OF THE CARDIORESPIRATORY CASE

1 HISTORY AND PHYSICAL EXAMINATION

PREDISPOSITIONS/PREDILECTIONS

AGE

- Congenital diseases usually appear in young animals, but it is not uncommon for mildly affected animals to live a normal life
- Respiratory tract infections tend to be more common in young unvaccinated animals
- Dilated cardiomyopathy (DCM) tends to occur in middle-aged dogs, 3–7 years of age, but younger and older animals may be affected
- Examples of diseases more common in older animals include:
  - Valvular endocardiosis
  - Chronic bronchitis
  - Idiopathic pulmonary fibrosis
  - Pulmonary neoplasia
  - Laryngeal paralysis
  - Hyperthyroidism in cats
  - Renal hypertension

SEX

Diseases more common in males
- Valvular endocardiosis
- Congenital AV valve dysplasia
- Idiopathic dilated cardiomyopathy (DCM)

Diseases more common in females
- Patent ductus arteriosus (PDA) (2:1)
- Addison's disease (hypoadrenocorticism)

BREED

Breed predispositions are invaluable for providing an initial differential list (see Appendix 1, pp. 185–6)

HISTORY

DETAILED CLINICAL HISTORY

- Identify the predominant cardiorespiratory clinical sign and its duration, severity and progression.
- Check vaccination and worming status.
- Check for a history of disease in the dam or sire.
- Evidence of contact with other animals, having been in an area of the UK where a particular condition is enzootic or having been abroad, may be important for respiratory diseases and parasitic diseases (lungworm or heartworm).
- The extent of lethargy, willingness to exercise, exercise tolerance and the presence of vomiting, diarrhoea, polydipsia and polyuria and appetite change should be noted.
- Check if there has been a long-standing

murmur present that would be suggestive of congenital heart disease or valvular endocardiosis.

- Any current or previous therapy and response to it should be noted.
- Check if the owners have noticed a putrid smell from the breath, which can be associated with foreign-body pneumonia.
- Check for evidence of trauma, even years prior to presentation, such as having been involved in a road traffic accident.
- Check for any history of scavenging or potential access to poisons such as paraquat and warfarin.
- Check if there is a previous history of neoplasms that have been surgically removed. If so, the histopathological identity of such tumours should be obtained.

BASIC PRINCIPLES IN TAKING A HISTORY

- Establish the primary reason the owner has presented the animal
- In difficult or complex cases this could take much longer than a routine consult time
- Ask non-leading questions
- Ask owners to describe what they actually saw (not their interpretation of what they think they saw)
- Do not diagnose conditions that do not explain the symptoms, e.g. the incidental heart murmur
- Do not find conditions that 'appear' to be present from blood work, radiographs, ECGs, etc. that do not fit logically with the symptoms
- Remember to check prior history, e.g. long-standing murmur, the forgotten mammary strip, the forgotten previous referral

CLINICAL EXAMINATION

GENERAL IMPRESSIONS/ OBSERVATION

- Debilitation and cachexia can be seen in dogs with congestive heart failure (particularly with dilated cardiomyopathy).
- Enlarged lymph nodes or palpable masses on the body surface or in the abdomen might suggest metastatic pulmonary neoplastic disease.
- Gross obesity severely compromises respiration and may be a precipitating cause of coughing in dogs with tracheal collapse. Obesity will also exacerbate coughing associated with pulmonary and cardiac disease.

SPECIFIC EXAMINATION OF THE CARDIORESPIRATORY SYSTEM

Mucosal colour
Mucosal colour is best evaluated from the gums or ocular mucosa (as opposed to the tongue)
- Pale
  - Low cardiac output (forward heart failure)
  - Shock (e.g. hypovolaemic)
  - Anaemia
- Congested ('flushed')
  - Venous congestion (right-sided congestive heart failure)
  - Polycythaemia
- Injected
  - Toxaemia/septicaemia (e.g. sepsis)

- Cyanosis
  - Check cranial and caudal membranes for a differential cyanosis, e.g. reverse-shunting PDA
  - Severe respiratory tract disease
  - Right-to-left shunting congenital cardiac defect (rare) – check for *polycythaemia*

Eyes

- Ocular discharges
  - Ophthalmic disease
  - Presence of a respiratory tract infection
- Examine retina for evidence of hypertension (intraocular/retinal haemorrhage)

Nose

- Nasal discharges (bi/unilateral)
  - Haemorrhagic (neoplasia, coagulation disorder)
  - Purulent (foreign body, bacterial, fungal)
- Depigmentation around the nares is often seen with fungal infection

Neck

- Jugular veins
  - Distension/pulsation: right-sided congestive heart failure, e.g. pericardial tamponade, tricuspid regurgitation, dysrhythmias (**Note**: the caudal vena cava should also be enlarged on chest radiographs)
  - In cats, pleural effusion of any cause can produce jugular distension
  - Check for enlarged thyroid lobes, e.g. hyperthyroidism
  - Feel the trachea for the dorsoventral flattening associated with tracheal collapse
  - Check tracheal sensitivity by compression (pinching) of the trachea to elicit coughing
  - Gentle inward lateral pressure on the larynx may exacerbate an inspiratory stridor in dogs with laryngeal paralysis (this is not useful in small-breed dogs)

Peripheral oedema

  - Cardiac disease (rare in small animals)
  - Hypoproteinaemia
  - Mediastinal masses
  - *Vena cava syndrome* (heartworm disease)
  - Angioedema
  - Vasculitis
  - Excessive fluid administration

Femoral pulses

- Check rate, rhythm and strength
  - In cats with aortic thromboembolism, either one or both pulses may not be palpable (in these cases also check the colour of the hind leg pads or nail bed)
  - Animals with a PDA usually have a very hyperdynamic (short and sharp) pulse, previously referred to as a 'waterhammer' pulse
  - A weak pulse may be found in dilated cardiomyopathy, but not necessarily with mitral valve disease
  - Dogs in congestive heart failure (CHF) usually have tachycardia, whereas those with respiratory disease are more likely to have a more normal rate, with sinus arrhythmia
  - Pulse deficit is defined as the absence of a palpable pulse following an audible heart beat
  - Pulse deficit may occur with premature beats or atrial fibrillation; typically there is a 50% pulse deficit in dogs with atrial fibrillation
  - *Pulsus paradoxus*: variation in pulse strength with respiration due to cardiac tamponade (pericardial effusion); the pulse is weaker during inspiration
  - *Pulsus alternans*: alternating pulse strength (not associated with an arrhythmia); seen when there is severe myocardial failure

Thoracic palpation

- Assess the strength of the apex beat
  - Increased in hypertrophic cardiomyopathy in cats
  - Increased with dilated cardiomyopathy and mitral valve disease in dogs
  - Reduced with pericardial or pleural effusion
- Check for displacement of apex beat, e.g. by a cranial thoracic or pulmonary mass
- Check for a precordial thrill (grade 5/6 or 6/6 heart murmurs)
- Check cats for reduced compliance of the cranial thoracic cage, which could indicate a cranial mediastinal mass

Abdominal palpation

- Assess liver size, the presence of masses.
- Ascites (which is a modified transudate) is often due to right-sided heart failure and less commonly due to obstruction of venous return or liver disease. To distinguish between these two possibilities, examine the jugulars for distension – if present then heart disease is almost certainly the cause of the ascites (pleural effusion can also produce jugular distension).

Respiratory pattern and respiratory rate

- The normal respiratory rate in dogs is <20/min and in cats is <40/min.
- The degree of tachypnoea or dyspnoea reflects the severity of disease.
- Care should be taken not to confuse tachypnoea with panting, which is physiological.

- In cats, mouth breathing is abnormal and implies the presence of dyspnoea.
- Hyperpnoea describes deep and purposeful respiration (sometimes seen with reverse-shunting heart defects).
- Inspiratory stridor suggests upper airway obstruction, such as laryngeal paralysis.
- Inspiratory dyspnoea indicates an airflow obstruction outside the thorax, e.g. laryngeal paralysis, cervical tracheal collapse.
- Expiratory dyspnoea tends to be an end-expiratory noise and is classically seen with thoracic tracheal collapse, chronic obstructive bronchial disease, intra-thoracic masses.
- Dyspnoea is best appreciated in non-tachypnoeic animals. When true dyspnoea is present it tends to prolong the associated phase of respiration, i.e. inspiratory dyspnoea will cause an increased inspiratory phase duration and vice versa.
- Orthopnoea, or breathing in sternal recumbency with the elbows abducted, is indicative of severe pulmonary changes or pleural effusion. These animals have minimal respiratory reserve and minor stress may be fatal.
- Pneumothorax is usually associated with an in-drawing of the intercostal spaces (into the 'vacuum') during inspiration.

> **Note:** Coughing in dogs may be due to cardiac or respiratory disease, usually the latter.

CHEST AUSCULTATION

Auscultation of the chest is best done with the animal standing.

> **Tip:** It is usually possible to stop a cat purring, by touching its nose with cotton wool soaked in spirit/alcohol.

RESPIRATORY AUSCULTATION

The international classification system for respiratory sounds is now widely used in veterinary medicine and is outlined below.

- *Wheezes* can be both inspiratory and expiratory and are associated with narrowing of airways.
  - An expiratory wheeze is typically associated with bronchoconstriction.
- *Rhonchi* are loud, low-pitched sounds associated with fast airflow through the larger airways. Consequently, they can appear in normal circumstances, such as after exercise. If there is upper airway obstruction the rhonchus noise is called *stridor* and is inspiratory.
- *Crackles*
  - Most commonly due to the re-opening of airways that have collapsed during expiration, and so are inspiratory.
  - Associated with bronchial disease (e.g. bronchitis, feline asthma), severe lung consolidation or intrathoracic airway collapse.
  - Can be heard when oedema fluid accumulates in the airways, usually only with advanced pulmonary oedema. (Note that interstitial oedema is not associated with this type of noise, which requires the mixing of air and fluid.)
- Additional sounds, such as râles and vesicular sounds, are no longer recognised respiratory terms, although bubbling and gurgling-type sounds can often be heard with bronchopneumonia.
- A combination of rhonchi, wheezes and crackles can be heard, giving complex sounds that may be difficult to identify.

Classification of abnormal (adventitious) respiratory sounds based on the American Thoracic Society Classification

Discontinuous sounds

Occur only during inspiration

- Crackles (associated with re-opening of collapsed airway)
  - Fine crackles
    - high pitch, low amplitude, short duration
  - Coarse crackles
    - low pitch, high amplitude, short duration

Continuous sounds

Can occur during inspiration or expiration

- Wheezes
  - Associated with airway narrowing
  - High pitch, variable amplitude and duration
- Rhonchi
  - Rapid air movement through larger airways
  - Low pitch, variable amplitude and duration
- Stridor
  - Upper airway (inspiratory)
- Stertor
  - Nasal passages and nasopharynx (inspiratory)

CARDIAC AUSCULTATION

The whole cardiac area (left and right) should be auscultated, and, additionally, in cats, the sternum, where gallops or murmurs can sometimes be heard best.

Area, audibility and position

- Note the area over which the heart can be heard. Is it larger than normal, suggesting the presence of cardiomegaly?
- Is the heart muffled, suggesting pericardial or pleural effusion?

- Is there displacement, e.g. by a thoracic or pulmonary mass?
- Any abnormal gut sounds, e.g. from a diaphragmatic hernia?

Rate and rhythm (Table 1.1)

Increased rate
- Heart failure, due to a compensatory sympathetic drive
- Physiological response, e.g. stress, excitement, fear
- Disease process, e.g. pyrexia, pain, anaemia, dehydration

Decreased rate
- Athletically fit dogs, e.g. working Border Collie
- Bradyarrhythmia
- Sinus bradycardia could be due to:
  - Hypothyroidism
  - Hyperkalaemia

- Hypothermia
- Elevated intracranial pressure
- Systemic disease (e.g. renal failure)
- Drugs (tranquillisers or antiarrhythmic drugs)

Rhythm
- *Sinus arrhythmia*
  - Heart rate that increases and decreases in a fairly regular rhythm often (but not always) with respiration
  - Can vary or be exaggerated, particularly in the presence of respiratory disease
- *Premature beats*
  - Can often be heard as an earlier than expected heart beat, which can create a 'tripping in the rhythm'
  - In some cases, the premature beat may have a reduced audibility and may be inaudible, thus it may sound like a

TABLE 1.1 A description of the heart rhythm that can be heard on auscultation, together with an indication of the heart rate with each rhythm and pulse strength

Rhythm	Rate	Pulse Regular
Regular		
• Sinus rhythm	Normal	Normal
• Sinus tachycardia	Fast	Normal/weak
• Sinus bradycardia	Slow	Normal/strong
• Ventricular tachycardia	Fast	Very weak
• Supraventricular tachycardia	Fast/very fast	Weak
• Heart block (may also hear atrial contraction A sounds)	Slow	Normal
Regularly Irregular		
• Sinus arrhythmia	Normal	Normal
Tripping in the Rhythm		
• Premature beats (VPCs or SVPCs)	Normal with extras	Deficit with prematures
• Sinus arrest/block	Normal with pauses	Normal with each beat
Chaotic		
• Atrial fibrillation	Variable	>50% pulse deficit
• Frequent premature beats (VPCs or SVPCs)	Variable	Pulse deficits associated with prematures

'dropped' or 'missed' beat and therefore mimic a sinus block/arrest
- *Atrial fibrillation* causes a chaotic rhythm (like 'slippers in a tumble dryer')
- *Complete heart block*
  - Usually a slow heart rate which is constant and does not vary
  - Compare with partial heart block or sinus bradycardia, which often have some variation in the rhythm
  - Virtually pathognomonic atrial contraction sounds (S4) may be heard (using the bell of the stethoscope) as a faster 'distant' sound

Murmurs

Murmurs are created due to vibration of structures within the heart, set in motion by abnormal, high-velocity blood flow and turbulence.

Timing
Systolic
Systolic murmurs are the most common and occur during ventricular contraction. These can be further classified as:
- Holosystolic – heart sounds can still be heard
  - May be associated with abnormal flow through the semilunar valves
- Pansystolic – murmur obscures the heart sounds
  - May be associated with AV incompetence and a ventricular septal defect.

Diastolic
Diastolic murmurs are rare in small animals.
- Most common cause is aortic regurgitation secondary to bacterial endocarditis
- Usually a very difficult murmur to hear, but it has a distinctive sound because of its timing (after the second heart sound) and it is decrescendo

Continuous
A continuous murmur is most commonly due to patent ductus arteriosus (PDA).

- Continuous because of the constantly present pressure difference between the aorta and pulmonary artery creating abnormally fast flow through the PDA
- Murmur is loudest during systole (when the pressure difference is greatest) and becomes quieter in diastole – i.e. it waxes and wanes during the cardiac cycle
- Previously referred to as a 'machinery' murmur

To and fro
A 'to and fro' murmur (which sounds like sawing wood) is due to the combination of a systolic murmur and a diastolic murmur:
- Subaortic stenosis with aortic regurgitation
- A ventricular septal defect with secondary aortic regurgitation
- Pulmonic stenosis with pulmonic regurgitation
- Can sometimes mimic a continuous murmur

Character
- *Harsh (ejection) murmurs* are associated with stenosis of the semilunar valves
  - Aortic stenosis
  - Pulmonic stenosis
- *Soft (or blowing) murmurs* are associated with valvular regurgitation
  - Mitral regurgitation
  - Tricuspid regurgitation
- Phonocardiography is able to classify these further as crescendo-decrescendo (stenosis murmurs) or constant intensity (regurgitant murmurs) but this is very difficult to appreciate on auscultation

Point of maximum intensity (PMI)
(Figure 1.1)
- Left heart base
  - Aortic stenosis
  - Pulmonic stenosis
  - PDA

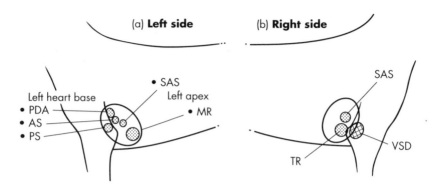

FIGURE 1.1(a,b)   The diagrams illustrate the point of maximum intensity (PMI) of cardiac murmurs due to various lesions. At the left heart base the murmurs of a PDA, AS and PS are heard maximally, at the left apex the murmur of mitral valve incompetence is heard best and over the 'mid-heart' area the murmur of SAS is heard. On the right thorax, the murmur due to tricuspid valve incompetence is heard over the mid to apical area, AS or SAS towards the right heart base and a VSD near the sternum and cranially

PDA: patent ductus arteriosus; AS: aortic stenosis; PS: pulmonic stenosis; MR: mitral regurgitation; SAS: subaortic stenosis; TR: tricuspid regurgitation; VSD: ventricular septal defect.

- Left heart apex
  - Mitral regurgitation
  - Some cases of subaortic aortic stenosis
- Right heart
  - Tricuspid regurgitation
  - Ventricular septal defect (often cranially near the sternum)
  - Aortic stenosis (nearer the base)

Intensity (Table 1.2)
Murmurs can be classified according to their loudness (intensity). Unfortunately, however, this does not necessarily reflect the severity of a lesion and there is variation in grading between operators.
- Murmurs that tend to increase in loudness with severity are caused by:
  - Aortic stenosis
  - Pulmonic stenosis
  - Mitral valve disease
- Murmurs whose loudness may not be proportional to severity are caused by:

  - Ventricular septal defect
  - Mitral regurgitation associated with dilated cardiomyopathy (DCM)
  - Murmurs with cardiomyopathies in cats

'Flow' or physiological murmurs tend to be fairly quiet (<grade 2 or 3) and may vary in intensity. These may occur with anaemia or fever or be normal in puppies.

Other heart sounds
- *Gallop sound (rhythm)* is the sound created by the addition of a third heart sound (S3 or S4) and is usually an indicator of heart disease in small animals.
- A *split S2* is most commonly as a result of delayed closure of the pulmonic valve, and may occur with pulmonic stenosis, a ventricular septal defect or pulmonary hypertension.
- A *systolic click* is a single clicking noise during systole. Its cause is unknown but may be due to mitral valve prolapse.

TABLE 1.2 Classification of murmurs based on intensity

Grade (out of 6)	Description	Simplified Grading System
1	Very quiet murmur that takes some time to find. Difficult to hear and usually only possible in a very quiet room.	Quiet
2	A very quiet murmur, but can usually be heard immediately.	Quiet
3	A murmur that is easy to hear, but not particularly loud.	Moderate
4	A loud murmur not associated with a palpable precordial thrill.	Moderate
5	A very loud murmur that is associated with a precordial thrill.	Loud
6	A precordial thrill and can be heard with the stethoscope lifted off the chest.	Loud

A summary of the essential questions to ask oneself during auscultation of the heart

1. Are the heart sounds louder or quieter than normal?
   • Does the apex beat feel stronger or weaker?
2. Is there a pulse for each heart beat?
   • Count heart and pulse rates
3. Is the rhythm:
   • Normal
   • Tripping
   • Chaotic
4. If there is a murmur:
   • Is the PMI left base, left apex or right?
   • Is it quiet, moderately loud or loud?
   • Is it continuous or not?
5. Is there a gallop sound?

TABLE 1.3 Differential diagnosis of cardiac versus respiratory disease

Clinical Sign	Cardiac Disease	Respiratory Disease
History		
Breathless	Yes	Yes
Cough	Yes	Yes
Exercise intolerance	Yes	Yes
Duration of cough	Short/medium	Chronic
Collapse	Common	Uncommon
Body condition	Normal/cachexia	Obese
Clinical Examination		
Mucosal colour	Pallor	Cyanosis
Apex beat	Increased or decreased	Normal
Pulse strength	Normal/decreased	Normal
Heart rate	Tachycardia	Normal
Sinus arrhythmia	Reduced/absent	Normal/pronounced
Ascites	With right CHF	If *cor pulmonale* (uncommon)
Ectopics	Likely	Rare
Auscultation		
Murmur	Present with MVD, often with other heart diseases	Could be present incidentally
Gallop sound	Cardiomyopathies most commonly	No
Large/loud heart	With cardiomegaly	Normal
Muffled heart	With pericardial disease	Normal
Pulmonary crackles	Airway oedema – rare	Airway disease – common

CHEST PERCUSSION

- The major use of chest percussion is to determine if thoracic lesions are asymmetric or if pneumothorax or pleural effusions are present.
- Pleural effusions may be detected if there is an obvious fluid-air interface. This is best appreciated in standing animals.

- Detecting asymmetric resonance gives guidelines as to which radiographic views to take. The resonance of the chest can be classified as normal, dull (pleural effusion, consolidated lung) or increased (pneumothorax, hyperinflated lung). The pitch of the resonant sound is directly related to the amount of air within the chest.

2 THORACIC RADIOGRAPHY

Thoracic radiography is an essential diagnostic aid in cardiac and respiratory medicine, however interpretation is dependent on the quality of the images obtained.

FACTORS INVOLVED IN OBTAINING GOOD-QUALITY RADIOGRAPHS

- Sufficiently powered X-ray unit, e.g. greater than 150 mA output
- Good quality films and screens; rare earth (fast) films and screens will help to reduce exposure time
- Automatic processing greatly reduces processing time and minimises processing faults
- A selection of restraining and positioning devices, such as sandbags, foam shapes (the wedge is most commonly used), ties, positioning troughs, is required

- Good centring and coning down with the light-beam diaphragm to minimise scatter radiation and thus improve contrast
- Although the use of grids will reduce scatter radiation, the increased exposure time required will increase movement blur so that grids are probably better avoided with low-output units
- Sedation or anaesthesia to minimise patient and/or respiratory movement and optimise positioning

TECHNIQUES IN THORACIC RADIOGRAPHY

This is not a discourse on radiographic technique, as there are many books on veterinary radiography that do this well, but the guidelines below may be of benefit to practitioners, as they highlight the common problems that the authors encounter from films submitted for interpretation.

MOST COMMON VETERINARY THORACIC RADIOGRAPHIC PROBLEMS

- *Poor processing* – primarily under-developing, because chemicals are not changed regularly

- *Recumbency atelectasis* – an artifact that mimics lung pathology
- *Inappropriate exposure* – under- or over-penetrated
- *Inadequate positioning* – rotated views, forelegs not pulled forward
- *Under-aerated lungs* – not taken during inspiration
- *Inadequate collimation or centring*

Film Processing

- Films that are *under-developed* appear flat and grey, lacking good black-and-white contrast, thus reducing detail. In a well-developed film, the directly exposed parts of the film (i.e. without body part) will be very black if the film is well processed

- The main reasons for under-developing are:
  - Not replacing the chemicals frequently enough
  - Not waiting for the chemical temperature to reach the correct level
  - If processing manually, not leaving the films in each tank for long enough
- It is a popular misconception that leaving the films in the developer for longer will balance out the problems of old or cool developer
- *Light fogging* will reduce film quality, and can be due to:
  - Light leakage under the darkroom door
  - A darkroom light bulb with too high a wattage (should be <25 W)
  - Having an incorrect darkroom light filter for the films used (e.g. green-sensitive film with an amber filter)
  - Forgetting to put the top on the film box

Tip: When the chemicals have been freshly changed, and the processor is up to temperature, radiograph a cassette directly using your usual middle-sized dog exposure. Develop the film and note how black the film is and keep it for future comparison. When there is a suspicion that radiographs are becoming flat due to under developing, take out the blank film and compare that with the black parts of the current film.

Recumbency atelectasis

- A problem primarily encountered in dogs
- Chest radiographs taken under sedation or anaesthesia
- In lateral recumbency there is atelectasis

of the dependent lung field, due to a combination of
  - hypoventilation because of sedation/anaesthesia
  - chest and heart weight on the dependent lungs
- Atelectasis is seen on DV (or VD) view and can be mistaken for lung pathology
- Extent of lung atelectasis is variable and from a mild increase in pulmonary density to almost the appearance of unilateral lung disease
- Associated mediastinal shift towards the collapsed lung(s), best appreciated as a shift in the heart position

Tip: The DV (or VD) view should be taken before the animal is placed in lateral recumbency. This is particularly important in an anaesthetised patient.

Radiographic exposure

- *High kV/low mAs* is preferred for thoracic radiographs
  - Lung detail is improved
  - Allows shorter exposure times (thereby reducing movement blur)
  - For feline chests a kV range of 58–66 is generally adequate
  - For canine chests a kV range of 70–90 is generally adequate (depending upon the size of dog)
- A *grid* should normally be used if the width of the thorax exceeds 12 cm. However, the increased exposure time required will increase movement blur and may be better avoided with low-output X-ray machines.
- Develop a *Technique Chart*. A technique chart reduces the frequency of over- and under-exposed films. Although there are a number of fairly complex methods in developing such a chart, a simple listing of the correct exposures found through trial and error for cats, small dogs,

medium dogs and large dogs will suffice in most instances. Simplifying the film/screen combinations used also helps.

Positioning

- The routine views for cardiac radiographs are DV and right lateral
- For respiratory radiographs, a DV and/or a VD view and both right and left laterals are useful
- A ready supply of sandbags and foam wedges all help in positioning the animal correctly
- When in lateral recumbency, the forelimbs should be pulled cranially out of the way so as not to obscure the cranial heart borders and cranial lung lobes, and a foam wedge should be placed under the sternum to prevent rotation of the body

DV or VD view

- Sternum and spine should be superimposed, indicating no rotation
- On cardiac radiographs the aortic line should be evident
- Respiratory radiographs are usually a slightly softer exposure to show lung detail better

Lateral view

- The costochondral junctions should be superimposed, indicating no rotation
- The caudal vena cava and cranial lobe vessels should be clearly evident
- Thrall's triangle (the triangle formed by the ventral border of vena cava, caudal border of heart and the diaphragm) should be large, indicating an inspiratory timed exposure. The distance along the ventral border of the caudal vena cava from the heart to diaphragm should be at least one intercostal space, but ideally nearer two.

Inspiratory views

These are most important *for assessing lung detail*.

- Exposures are best taken *during* inspiration (if not manually inflated)
- In respiratory cases in *dogs*, it is often useful to take X-rays under GA in order to inflate the lungs during the exposure (to normal tidal volume). This maximises the air-to-soft-tissue contrast detail and also minimises motion blur. **Note:** manual lung inflation is not necessary in cats and should not be performed
- Expiratory timed exposures can also give the optical illusion of cardiomegaly – use the vertebral heart score to assess heart size if in doubt
- Both inspiratory and expiratory views are useful when radiographing for
  ○ Tracheal collapse in dogs
  ○ Asthma in cats

Collimation and radiation safety

- If chemical restraint is adequate (See Appendix 7, pp. 193–4), animals should rarely need to be held for thoracic radiographs.
- All radiographs should be centred over the area of interest and collimated down to it. This reduces scatter and improves film quality.

ASSESSMENT OF THORACIC RADIOGRAPHS FOR QUALITY

- X-rays should be viewed in a consistent manner:
  ○ Lateral radiographs are usually placed with the animal's head to the viewer's left
  ○ DV (or VD) radiograph with the animal's right side to the viewer's left.
- When examining a film, note the position, the normality or abnormality for each structure.

- In normal animals, the predominant pattern in the lung is due to the pulmonary vessels, while the additional *greyness* of the pattern is attributed to the lung parenchyma.
- Marginal over- or under-exposure can result in marked changes in radiographic detail which can significantly affect interpretation and reduce diagnostic value, if the pathological changes are subtle.
- A thoracic radiograph with poor lung inflation is characterised by increased soft tissue density (i.e. lacking air contrast), making structures indistinct and potentially leading to over-interpretation of the density (e.g. giving the illusion of an interstitial pattern).
- An over-inflated film is characterised by a flattened diaphragm.

ASSESSMENT OF THE RESPIRATORY SYSTEM

The lung pattern changes in response to both respiratory and cardiac diseases, but from the assessment of the cardiac silhouette the primary source of the problem should be identified.

- The normal lung pattern consists primarily of the pulmonary vasculature. Vessels are mostly seen adjacent to bronchi, with the arteries dorsal (on the lateral view) and lateral (on the VD/DV view) to the adjacent bronchus. Veins are ventral and medial to the bronchi respectively.
- Pulmonary vessels appear as lines that taper and branch towards the periphery or as solid circular shadows if viewed end-on.
- The bronchi are seen because they are delineated by the adjacent blood vessels and the air within the bronchi. The vascular pattern is more prominent in the cat.
- The rest of the normal lung pattern is presumed to represent the lung parenchyma. This pattern is linear, but whereas the pulmonary vasculature, particularly in the cat, spreads out towards the lung periphery, the interstitial pattern is more haphazard giving a reticulated appearance to the lung field.

VASCULAR PATTERN

This is the predominant density in normal lung. Note that abnormal vascular patterns are difficult to appreciate and are dependent on film quality and respiratory timing.

Over-circulation (hypervascularity)
- The vessels appear 'fatter' than normal (over-circulated or congested) and extend further into the periphery
- Left-to-right cardiac shunt (VSD, PDA)

Passive pulmonary congestion
- The pulmonary veins are 'fatter', and sometimes denser, than their associated arteries as they become congested
- Left-sided heart failure

Under-circulation (hypovascularity)
The vessels appear thinner than normal (under-circulated) and seem reduced in number in the periphery. This effect is often enhanced by a concurrent hyper-inflation of the lung to compensate for the reduced perfusion.
- Hypovolaemia/dehydration
- Shock
- Hypoadrenocorticism
- Pulmonic stenosis
- Right-to-left shunt

Distended and tortuous vessels

- Pulmonary thromboembolism
- Pulmonary hypertension
- Heartworm disease (dirofilariasis)

BRONCHIAL PATTERN

Bronchial walls are not normally visible, but can be appreciated coursing between the associated artery and vein. When there is disease involving the bronchi (peribronchial or bronchial), the bronchial walls are seen on radiograph as parallel lines ('tramlines'). Thickened bronchial walls seen from an end-on view will appear as rings ('doughnuts'). An end-on bronchus may occasionally be seen with its associated vessel ('signet ring'). In chronic airway disease the bronchi often become dilated (tubular or saccular bronchiectasis).

Causes of bronchial-wall thickening

- Age-related change in dogs
- Allergic airway diseases, e.g. feline asthma, pulmonary infiltrate with eosinophilia (PIE)
- Inflammatory diseases (bronchitis, bacterial, viral, fungal)
- Parasitic diseases (infection with *Angiostrongylus, Crenosoma, Oslerus, Aelurostrongylus, Dirofiliaria, Toxoplasma*)
- Bronchial carcinoma
- Inhalational irritants

Causes of bronchial-wall mineralisation

- Age-related change
- Hyperadrenocorticism
- Hyperparathyroidism

ALVEOLAR PATTERN

Alveoli and bronchioles are not normally visible. When the alveoli fill with fluid (e.g. oedema, blood, exudate) or cellular infiltrate or collapse, they form soft tissue densities, thus outlining the air-filled bronchioles (air bronchograms). There is an associated loss of the vascular walls and bronchial walls.

Causes of an alveolar pattern

- Cardiogenic pulmonary oedema (left-sided congestive heart failure)
  - In dogs: Often perihilar and bilaterally symmetrical, but can affect the right lung fields more that the left, and can be diffuse
  - In cats: Often diffuse and more ventral, but can be patchy
- Non-cardiogenic pulmonary oedema – often symmetrical and affecting the caudal lobes most
  - Acute dyspnoea due to obstructive airway disease
  - Neurogenic: seizures, brain trauma, hypoglycaemia, electrocution
  - I/v fluid overload
  - Lymphatic obstruction
  - Toxins
  - Drowning
  - Paraquat poisoning
  - Smoke inhalation
  - Shock
  - DIC
  - Heat stroke
  - Hypoalbuminaemia
- Haemorrhage
  - Pulmonary contusion – tends to be localised to site of trauma
  - Lungworm disease – tends to affect caudal dorsal lung field
  - Lung lobe torsion – affects a single lung lobe, commonly a middle or cranial lobe
- Bronchopneumonia
  - FB pneumonia commonly affects right or left caudal lobe
  - Aspiration (inhalation) pneumonia tends to affect ventral lobes
  - Eosinophilic pneumonia

- Pneumonitis
- Bronchial obstruction (FB, extra- or intraluminal mass)
- Pulmonary infarct (from pulmonary thromboembolism) – tends to affect peripheral caudal dorsal lung
- Bronchoalveolar carcinoma
- Atelectasis or collapse (recumbency artifact, pneumothorax)

INTERSTITIAL PATTERN

The normal interstitium (alveolar walls and supporting tissue) gives the background hazy/grey appearance to the lung. When disease affects the interstitium it becomes thickened and therefore more visible as a fine linear or reticular mesh-like pattern. It differs from the vascular pattern in not following any particular direction. The pattern it creates is sometimes described as 'lace-like' or 'honeycomb'. An interstitial pattern sometimes obscures the vessels towards their periphery.

- Possibly a common, non-specific age-related change
- Artifact
  - Under-penetrated film
  - Under-aerated (expiratory) film
- Obesity
- Pulmonary oedema (before progressing to alveolar oedema)
- Interstitial pneumonia
- Idiopathic pulmonary fibrosis
- *Pneumocystis carinii* pneumonia
- Eosinophilic pneumonia
- Paraquat poisoning
- Neoplasia: lymphoma, bronchoalveolar carcinoma, widespread metastatic disease
- Lungworm disease
- Fungal disease (coccidiomycosis, histoplasmosis)

CAVITATORY LESIONS

- Cysts, bullae, blebs (congenital or acquired)
- Abscess
- Trauma
- Granuloma
- Neoplasia (primary)
- Bronchial obstruction – pneumatocoele

PLEURAL EFFUSION AND PNEUMOTHORAX

- The presence of pleural effusion or pneumothorax is assessed. With mild effusions the radiographs should be inspected for subtle lobe-fissure lines, particularly on the ventrodorsal views.
- The position and width of the mediastinum are noted. On the VD or DV view the cranial mediastinum generally should not be wider than the vertebrae.
- Free air in the mediastinum will cause the structures within it to be highlighted (arteries, veins, oesophagus).
- Air in the oesophagus can be appreciated as an irregular, thin, radiopaque line at its dorsal and ventral aspects, on the lateral view.
- The oesophagus overlies the trachea, and any air within the oesophagus highlights the dorsal tracheal wall ('stripe' sign). In the conscious animal no air should be apparent within the oesophagus, but it is commonly found under general anaesthesia and sedation.
- From a thorough examination of good-quality radiographs it should be possible to determine the degree of cardiac involvement in the lung changes seen (vascular congestion and pulmonary oedema), if the changes are primarily due to respiratory disease, and to classify the predominant lung and airway pattern.

ASSESSMENT OF THE CARDIOVASCULAR SYSTEM

Despite the advent of Doppler echocardiography, thoracic radiography remains the optimal diagnostic procedure for the assessment of the degree of volume load (pulmonary congestion or oedema). Good-quality thoracic radiographs are superior to auscultation for the detection of pulmonary oedema and assessment of the degree of congestion (and thus the appropriate dose of diuretics).

NORMAL HEART SIZE AND SHAPE

Dog

In the dog there is marked breed variation, and the clinician's ability to assess heart size and shape often depends on experience. Even then, the accuracy of radiography for the diagnosis of cardiomegaly has been questioned. Deep, narrow-chested dogs (Greyhound, setters, etc.) have a very upright heart, with little sternal contact. In contrast, broad-chested dogs (Labrador, Bull Terrier, etc.) can have a heart that appears almost to lie on the sternum, with the appearance of increased sternal contact.

Lateral view
- Height should not exceed two thirds of the depth of the thorax.
- Width is approximately 2.5–3.5 rib spaces.
- Cardiac size on this view can be assessed by measuring the apicobasilar heart length and the width of the heart at right angles to this line at its widest point. The combined sum of these two measurements (the Vertebral Heart Scale) should normally be 8.5–10.5 vertebrae, starting from the fourth thoracic vertebra.

- Distal portion of the trachea should run fairly parallel to the sternum, and its ventral border often runs in a gentle arcing curve to the caudal border of the heart.
- There should be a fairly distinct caudal waist, created by the caudal border of the heart and the ventral border of the caudal lobe pulmonary vessels.

Dorsoventral view
- Heart appears as an inverted D, with a fairly straight edge to the left heart border.
- Width should not exceed two thirds of the thorax.
- Length should lie between the third and eighth ribs.
- The silhouette of the heart can be viewed as a clock face on the DV view (Figure 2.1). Although this is a very useful analogy to use, displacement of the cardiac apex can distort this analogy. For example, an enlarged left ventricle that pushes the apex to the right may be mistaken as right ventricular enlargement if using the clock-face analogy. It is therefore important to establish where the cardiac apex is, although this is often difficult when there is gross cardiomegaly.

Cat

In the cat, the heart is fairly uniform in size and position between breeds. Obese cats can have an apparent cardiomegaly.

Lateral view
- The apicobasilar angle to the sternum is approximately 45°
- The apicobasilar length of the heart is not greater than two thirds the internal depth of the thorax
- The width (measured at right angles to the apicobasilar heart line) should not exceed two rib spaces

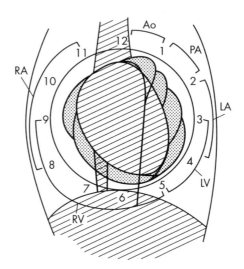

FIGURE 2.1 Schematic diagram illustrating how the cardiac silhouette on a DV thoracic radiograph can be viewed as a 'clock face'.

- At 12–1 o'clock, a bulge in the aortic arch may be evident with aortic stenosis or a patent ductus arteriosus. Note that the left lateral edge of the descending aorta is usually evident on a good exposure and this can be seen to run to a bulge in the aortic arch.
- At 1–2 o'clock, a bulge in the pulmonary artery may be evident, e.g. due to pulmonic stenosis, patent ductus arteriosus or pulmonary hypertension.
- At 2–4 o'clock, a smooth bulge due to enlargement of the left auricle can be seen, e.g. secondary to mitral endocardiosis or a VSD.
- At 3–5 o'clock, rounding of the heart border may be associated with left ventricular enlargement.
- At 5–9 o'clock, rounding of the heart border may be seen with right ventricular enlargement.
- At 8–11 o'clock, a bulge may be seen due to right atrial enlargement.

Key: Ao – aorta, PA – pulmonary artery, LA – left auricle, LV – left ventricle, RV – right ventricle, RA – right atrium.

Dorsoventral view
- The width of the heart does not exceed two thirds the internal width of the chest
- The Vertebral Heart Scale width of the normal heart on the DV view should be <4

ABNORMAL HEART SIZE AND SHAPE

- Generalised cardiomegaly
  - Breed variation
  - Dilated cardiomyopathy
  - Long standing mitral valve disease

- o Right atrial enlargement associated with tricuspid dysplasia
- o Pericardial effusion
- Microcardia
  - o Hypovolaemia
  - o Addison's disease

SIGNS OF LEFT-SIDED HEART ENLARGEMENT

Left atrial enlargement

Thoracic radiographs are particularly sensitive in detecting left atrial enlargement.

Lateral view

- Straightening of the caudal border of the heart and loss of the caudal waist (as this area is filled by the enlarging left atrium).
- Elevation of the distal trachea, which becomes more parallel to the spine.
- Elevation of the mainstem bronchi with usually the left caudal mainstem bronchus being elevated above the right. This appears as a splitting of the mainstem bronchi (this may artifactually occur when the chest positioning is rotated).

Dorsoventral view

- Mild to marked bulging of the cardiac silhouette at the 2–4 o'clock position (**Note:** This is in fact the left auricle rather than the atrium). In the cat, the bulge can be a distinct shoulder, more towards the 2–3 o'clock position.
- In dogs, the caudal lobe bronchi can appear to be displaced or pushed laterally by the enlarged atrium between them.

Left ventricular enlargement

Radiographs are fairly insensitive at detecting left ventricular enlargement.

Lateral view

- There may be rounding of the caudal border with increased contact with the diaphragm

- The caudal vena cava may appear horizontal, or even elevated (i.e. run 'uphill' to the heart)

Dorsoventral view

- The left border may become more rounded at the 3–5 o'clock position
- The apex may appear midline or even pushed over to the right

Signs of aortic arch enlargement

- On the lateral view, the aortic arch may bulge into the cranial mediastinum. This may be normal in old cats and has been referred to as a 'redundant' aorta.
- On the DV view, a bulging aorta may be evident at the 12–1 o'clock position. Its position can be confirmed by following the left lateral edge of the descending aorta.

Causes of an aortic bulge

- Aortic stenosis – post-stenotic bulge
- Patent ductus arteriosus

SIGNS OF RIGHT HEART ENLARGEMENT

Right atrium

Lateral view

The cranial border of the heart may appear more rounded. In some cases severe enlargement may cause elevation of the trachea just proximal to its bifurcation. Very marked enlargement can mimic the globoid heart of pericardial effusion.

Dorsoventral view

There is often a bulge at the 8–11 o'clock position.

Right ventricle

Lateral view

- There may be increased sternal contact (allowing for breed variation) and rounding of the cranial heart border
- Marked right ventricular hypertrophy

may cause the apex of the heart to lift off the sternum and tip up towards the diaphragm

Dorsoventral view
- The right heart border is rounded at the 5–9 o'clock position
- The cardiac apex may be pushed more towards the left

Caudal vena cava
- Increase in diameter (best seen on the lateral view)
  - May be associated with signs of right-sided congestive failure
  - **Note:** Also check for hepatic venous congestion

Pulmonary artery enlargement
Lateral view
- There may be an enlargement of the craniodorsal heart border, towards the cranial mediastinum
- A semi-circular shadow may appear to overlie the distal trachea, due to a post-stenotic bulge, often referred to as a 'cap'

Dorsoventral view
- There may be a bulge at the 1–2 o'clock position

Causes of a pulmonary artery bulge
- Pulmonic stenosis – post-stenotic bulge
- Patent ductus arteriosus
- Pulmonary artery hypertension

CONGESTIVE HEART FAILURE

Radiographic signs of left-sided congestive heart failure

Note: Left-sided congestive failure should be associated with the appropriate left heart enlargement, particularly left atrial enlargement, except in some acute presentations (e.g. ruptured *chordae tendineae* and acute DCM).

- With *pulmonary venous congestion* the veins appear wider than their associated arteries (best seen in the cranial lung lobes). The veins may be greater than 75% of the width of the dorsal portion of the third rib.
- With *pulmonary oedema* there is often a mixed interstitial and alveolar pattern. Initially, in dogs, the appearance is of indistinct, fluffy, 'cotton-wool' or 'cloud-like' soft tissue densities around the hilus. This becomes more widespread with severe oedema. In cats, the distribution of oedema is more widespread and diffuse, and needs to be differentiated from feline asthma, neoplasia and aelurostrongylosis.

Common causes of left-sided congestive heart failure
- Mitral valve endocardiosis
- Dilated cardiomyopathy
- Feline cardiomyopathies
- Congenital mitral valve dysplasia
- Ventricular septal defect
- Patent ductus arteriosus
- Aortic stenosis with mitral valve incompetence (rare)

Radiographic signs of right-sided congestive heart failure

> **Note:** Right sided congestive failure should be associated with the appropriate right heart enlargement.

- The caudal vena cava may appear 'fat', often greater than the diameter of the aorta. The cranial vena cava is sometimes evident on the DV view to the right of the mediastinum
- Hepatomegaly
- Ascites
- Pleural effusion

Common causes of right-sided congestive heart failure
- Pericardial effusion
- Tricuspid endocardiosis
- Congenital tricuspid valve dysplasia
- Pulmonic stenosis with tricuspid valve incompetence
- Caval syndrome (heartworm disease)
- *Cor pulmonale*

Common causes of left- and right-sided failure
- Dilated cardiomyopathy
- Feline cardiomyopathies

ANGIOGRAPHY

- Angiocardiography has mostly been superseded by Doppler echocardiography, but still finds a use in specialist centres in association with interventional procedures (e.g. balloon pulmonary valvuloplasty, patent ductus arteriosus occlusion).
- Non-selective angiography is an easy procedure to perform, with minimal costs involved, but is less useful. It can be useful in detecting reverse (right-to-left) shunting defects, although echocontrast is an alternative option.
- Contrast medium can be introduced into a heart chamber by catheterisation (direct, selective) or through a peripheral vein, such as the jugular (indirect, non-selective).

3 ELECTROCARDIOGRAPHY

Electrocardiography should be done in the light of a thorough clinical examination of the cardiovascular system, paying particular attention to heart rate and rhythm, pulse rate and identification of pulse deficits if present.

USES OF ELECTROCARDIOGRAPHY

- Arrhythmias
  - Definitive diagnosis of an irregular heart rhythm in cardiac and non-cardiac cases
  - Monitoring
    - In the perianaesthetic period
    - After road traffic accidents (traumatic myocarditis)
    - In animals with gastric dilation/volvulus, pancreatitis, pyometra
    - During pericardiocentesis
- Electrolyte disturbances
  - Hyperkalaemia
    - Addison's disease
    - Acute renal failure
    - Diabetic ketoacidosis
  - Hypokalaemia
  - Hypercalcaemia
- Cardiac chamber enlargement
- Pericardial effusion
- Drug effects – e.g. digitalis toxicity, quinidine, propranolol
- Myocardial ischaemia and fibrosis
- Assessment of response to treatment (serial ECGs)

THE ELECTROCARDIOGRAPH (ECG)

For a useful beginner's guide to small animal electrocardiography, the reader is referred to Martin (2000)

- An *electrocardiograph* (ECG machine) is a voltmeter (or galvanometer) that records the changing electrical activity of the heart between positive and negative electrodes. *Electrocardiography* is the process of recording these electrical changes.
- Electrodes are placed on the legs of the animal – referred to as a *body surface limb ECG recording*.

CARDIAC ELECTROPHYSIOLOGY

- Cardiac cells have basically two characteristic transmembrane action potentials, those of *myocardial* cells and those of *pacemaker* cells.
- *Pacemaker cells* differ from myocardial cells in that they possess *automaticity*, i.e. the resting membrane potential is not stable but gradually rises until it reaches a threshold level and an action potential is triggered.

- *Myocardial cells* do not possess automaticity except when abnormal, resulting in ectopic depolarisations – termed *abnormal automaticity.*
- The *sino-atrial node (SAN)* is the *dominant pacemaker* tissue in the heart because its intrinsic rate is faster than that of other pacemaker cells.
- Other pacemaker cells exist: *A V node,* the *Bundle of His, bundle branches, Purkinje fibres.* These cells are prevented from acting as pacemakers, however, because of the faster rate of the SAN and *overdrive suppression* by the dominant pacemaker (SAN).
- The intrinsic heart rate is dictated by the rate of diastolic depolarisation of pacemaker cells in the SA node. This rate is altered by the balance of autonomic tone, increased by sympathetic stimulation and decreased by parasympathetic stimulation.
- Imbalances in autonomic tone may be physiological or stress related.

FORMATION OF THE P-QRS-T COMPLEX

- All cells within the heart have the ability to generate their own electrical activity, but the *sinoatrial (SA) node* is the fastest to do so and is therefore the rate controller, termed the *pacemaker.*
- Rate of the SA node is influenced by the balance in autonomic tone, i.e. the *sympathetic* (increases rate) and *parasympathetic* (decreases rate) systems.
- The SA node initiates the electrical discharge for each cardiac cycle.
- Depolarization spreads through the atrial muscle cells, then spreads through the *atrioventricular (AV) node.*
- Conduction passes through the AV ring (from the atria into the ventricles), through a narrow pathway called the *Bundle of His,* then divides in the ven-

tricular septum into *left and right bundle branches.* The left bundle branch divides into *anterior and posterior fascicles.*
- The conduction tissue spreads into the myocardium as very fine branches called *Purkinje fibres.*

Isoelectric line

An isolectric line is a line on an ECG that results when there is no potential difference across the heart, i.e. all cells are in the resting phase.

P wave

- When the pacemaker cells trigger an impulse, a wave of excitation is transmitted across the atria, resulting in a potential difference between the area of cells that are depolarised first and the area of cells that have not yet been stimulated. This is recorded as a deflection on the ECG.
- When all the cells of both atria are depolarised, there will be no potential difference, current flow will cease and the pen of the ECG recorder will return to the isoelectric line.

PR interval

- This is the interval from the start of the P wave to the start of the QRS complex (strictly therefore a PQ interval). Much of the PR interval is produced by the delay in conduction through the AV node.

QRS complex

- This waveform represents depolarisation of the ventricular myocardial mass.
- Depolarisation begins in the septum, creating a small summation vector in a direction *away* from the positive electrode and recorded on the ECG as a small downward, or *negative,* deflection. This *first* negative deflection on an ECG is defined as the Q *wave.*
- The wave of excitation then spreading throughout the bulk of the ventricular

myocardium causes a large potential difference (greater mass of tissue), and therefore a larger current, in the general direction of the positive electrode. This is seen as a large *positive* deflection on the ECG. This *first* positive deflection (in the QRS complex) is defined as the *R wave*.

- Finally the remaining basilar parts of both ventricles and septum are depolarised, creating a small current of flow away from the positive electrode and a small *negative* deflection on the ECG. The *first* negative deflection *after the R wave* is defined as the *S wave*.

S-T Segment

- This period coincides with the plateau phase of the action potential, prior to repolarisation.
- This is the period from the end of the S wave (J point) to the start of the *T wave*.

T wave

- Represents repolarisation of the ventricular myocardium
- In the dog and cat, the direction of the T wave is variable
- The T wave can be positive, negative or biphasic, and its direction is not significant

RECORDING AN ELECTROCARDIOGRAM

LEAD SYSTEMS

- There are three bipolar leads: I, II and III; and three augmented unipolar leads: aVR, aVL and aVF.
- Recordings can also be made by the use of unipolar precordial *chest leads*. The chest leads can be useful in detecting ventricular enlargement, bundle-branch block, myocardial infarction and visualising P waves that are small in the limb leads.

PROCEDURE FOR RECORDING OF AN ECG

Positioning

- Right lateral recumbency is the standard position in the dog. However, it has been shown that restraint of cats in sternal recumbency makes little difference to complex amplitudes.
- If the recording of arrhythmias is the only concern or the animal is in severe respiratory distress, then any comfortable position may be adopted.
- It is preferable not to use any form of chemical restraint as it may interfere with the heart rhythm and mask or produce arrhythmias.

Chemical restraint for electrocardiography

- All sedative and tranquilliser drugs have a variable effect on the heart and/or autonomic tone and therefore change the rate and rhythm of the heart directly or through effects upon autonomic tone.
- If an ECG is performed to diagnose an arrhythmia heard on auscultation, then use of chemical restraint is likely to change the rhythm – thus a *representative* ECG is not obtained.
- If chemical restraint cannot be avoided, then, based upon physical examination, determine the heart *and* pulse rates and rhythm, before *and* after sedation – any differences should be taken into account when interpreting the ECG.

Electrical contact

- Electrode leads attached by: crocodile clips, paediatric limb electrodes or adhesive electrodes.

- Sites for placement of the electrodes:
  - Caudal and proximal to the elbows and just above the patellar ligaments.
  - Flexor angle of the elbow or distal to the elbow caudally and the flexor angle of the hock.
- The electrodes should be placed directly onto a loose fold of skin ensuring as much contact as possible. The hair should be parted to allow proper contact.
- Contact is improved by the use of a conductive medium, e.g. conductive ECG gel or spirit.

ARTIFACTS

Artifacts mask the ECG recording or mimic ECG activity – producing an artifact-free tracing is of paramount importance.

Electrical interference

Electrical interference appears as fine, rapid and regular movements on the baseline of the ECG recording. They are often associated with interference due to electrical lines (electromagnetic) within the room in which the recording is being made. They can be transmitted by the person restraining the animal who acts as an aerial or through the power line of the ECG machine. The fine deflections usually occur at a rate of 50/sec (60/sec in America).

To correct this problem:

- Ensure the clip-to-skin connections are good and are insulated (isolated) – poor connections will permit electrical interference to manifest itself
- Ensure the animal is insulated from the surface by placing a rug under it
- Ensure the ECG machine is earthed (to the building), or try not to run on the mains supply but on battery
- Try insulating the handlers from the dog by having them wear gloves

Muscle tremor artifact

Muscle tremor can look similar to electrical interference, but the fine deflections in this instance are not regular but random. It can be produced by the animal trembling or shaking or by trying to record the ECG in a standing animal. Purring in a cat will also result in baseline 'trembling'!

To correct this problem:

- Ensure the limbs are relaxed and supported
- Find a position in which the animal will relax best – preferably not standing
- Try holding the limbs to minimise the tremor
- To stop cats purring: Dab a little spirit on the cat's nose using cotton wool

Movement artifact

Movement artifact is a more exaggerated form of tremor artifact, but in this case the deflections are not fine but variable and large. The stylus moves up and down the paper. It can be associated with respiratory movement or the animal moving or struggling. Correction of this is similar to tremor artifact.

- Try to get the animal to relax and remain still
- Ensure the ECG cables are not moving with movement of the animal, e.g. respiratory movement, or because the clips are not stable and secure.

Incorrectly placed electrodes

This may result in inverted complexes or bizarre mean electrical axis.

> **Tip:** P waves are nearly always positive in leads I, II and III. Double check the position of the ECG cables.

THE NORMAL ECG

Refer to the table of normal values and mean electrical axis (MEA) (Table 3.1).
- Note that a normal ECG does not rule out:
  - *Heart enlargement*, as the vectors in the frontal plane may be within normal limits or the complex amplitudes may be damped by fluid (pericardial,

TABLE 3.1   Normal ECG values for dogs and cats (Tilley 1992)

Parameter	Canine	Normal Value	Feline	Normal Value
Rate	Adult	70–160	Adult	120–240
	Giant breeds	60–140	Average rate	~190–200
	Toy breeds	70–180		
	Puppy	70–220		
P Wave Duration	Maximum	0.04 sec	Maximum	0.04 sec
	Giant breeds maximum	0.05 sec		
P Wave Amplitude	Maximum	0.4 mV	Maximum	0.2 mV
P-R Interval	Range	0.06–0.13 sec	Range	0.05–0.09 sec
QRS Duration	Maximum	0.05 sec	Maximum	0.04 sec
	Large breeds maximum	0.06 sec		
R Wave Amplitude	Maximum	2.5 mV	Maximum	0.9 mV
	Large breeds maximum	2.0 mV		
S-T Segment	Maximum depression	0.2 mV	No depression	n/a
	Maximum elevation	0.15 mV	No elevation	n/a
T Wave	Can be positive, negative or biphasic	<1/4 of R wave amplitude	Can be positive, negative or biphasic	
			Maximum	0.3 mV
Q-T Interval	Range at normal heart rate	0.15–0.25 sec	Range at normal heart rate	0.12–0.18 sec
Mean Electrical Axis	Range	+40° to +100°	Range	0 to +160°

Note: Some measurements differ for deep-chested dogs less than two years of age.

pleural or ascitic) or some pulmonary diseases and obesity
  ○ *Arrhythmias*, as they might not be present at the time of recording
- Measurements that are slightly abnormal may be normal for that individual
- Thin animals may have larger amplitudes
- Young animals (<12 months) often have a large Q wave

NORMAL RHYTHMS

Sinus rhythm

- Arises from the SA node, producing a normal P wave followed by normal QRS and T waves
- The rhythm is constant and regular
- The rate is within normal for the breed

Clinical findings

- There are regular heart sounds on auscultation, with a pulse for each heart beat at a rate which is normal for age, breed and species.

Sinus arrhythmia

- Arises from the SA node
- Rate varies (increases and decreases) regularly
- Occurs as a result of vagal tone
- Often synchronous with respiration
- Common in dogs and a good indicator of the absence of increased sympathetic drive, such as occurs in heart failure
- Uncommon in the cat (sinus rhythm is more common)

Clinical findings

- The heart rhythm varies with some regularity – increasing and decreasing in rate with a pulse for every heartbeat.

Wandering pacemaker

- Occurs as a result of the dominant pacemaker shifting from the SA node to other pacemaker cells with a high intrinsic rate within the atria
- Results in P waves that vary in amplitude and direction (i.e. positive, negative or biphasic)
- Usually a regular variation
- May be associated with high vagal tone
- More common in the dog

THE ABNORMAL ECG

CHANGES INDICATIVE OF CHAMBER ENLARGEMENT

LA enlargement

- P wave prolonged (dog and cat: >0.04 sec) and/or notched (referred to as *P-mitrale*, as LA enlargement is often associated with mitral valve disease)
- Occurs as a result of asynchronous depolarisation of the right and left atria, the latter being last to do so

Note: Giant breeds may have normally prolonged P waves (0.05 sec)

RA enlargement

- P wave of increased amplitude (dog: >0.4 mV; cat: >0.2 mV), especially leads II and III, and aVF
- Referred to as *P-pulmonale*, as RA enlargement may be associated with *cor pulmonale*

LV enlargement

- Tall R waves in leads II and III and aVF (dog: >2.5 mV; cat: >0.9 mV)
- R wave in lead I greater than lead II or aVF (may be associated with hypertrophy)

- Increased R waves in I, II and III may be associated with dilation
- QRS duration prolonged (dog: >0.05 sec; cat: >0.04 sec)
- S-T segment sagging/coving
- MEA shifted to the left (dog: <+40°; cat: <0°)

Note: Need to differentiate from left bundle branch block and anterior fascicular block.

RV enlargement

- Deep S waves in leads I, II, III and aVF
- MEA shifted to the right (dog: >+100°; cat: >+160°)

Note: Need to differentiate from right bundle branch block.

ARRHYTHMIAS

- Literally means absence of rhythm; dysrhythmia is a synonymous term
- Arrhythmias that are essentially slow are referred to as *bradyarrhythmias*, and those that are fast as *tachyarrhythmias*

Note: The reader is referred to Chapter 7 for treatment of arrhythmias.

A representative rhythm strip

- Ensure that the ECG recording obtained is representative of the physical examination findings.
- If an arrhythmia heard on auscultation is not revealed on the ECG rhythm strip, then simultaneously auscultate the animal whilst continuing to run the ECG recording. It might be that the abnormality is only intermittently present, in which case continue to auscultate the animal until the arrhythmia is heard and then captured on ECG.

ABNORMALITIES IN RATE

Sinus bradycardia

- Normal P-QRS-T complexes at a slower rate than normal

Clinical findings

- The heart rate is slower than normal for age and breed, with a pulse for every heart beat.

Sinus tachycardia

- Normal P-QRS-T complexes at a faster rate than normal
- Very common in the cat

Clinical findings

- The heart rate is faster than normal for age and breed, with a pulse for every heart beat.

ABNORMALITIES IN CONDUCTION

Sinus arrest/block

- Failure of pacemaker to discharge results in a pause with no P-QRS-T complex
- If pause is twice R-R interval, it suggests block
- If pause is greater than twice R-R interval, it suggests arrest
- Long periods of arrest are usually followed by escape complexes

Clinical findings

- A silent pause in the heart rhythm will be appreciated on auscultation (with no palpable pulse). It will sound like the heart has momentarily stopped.

Sick sinus syndrome (sinus node dysfunction)

- A term for a number of abnormalities of the SA node, including severe sinus bradycardia and severe SA block/arrest

- Many of these cases also have episodes of supraventricular tachycardias, termed *bradycardia-tachycardia syndrome*
- It is characteristic of this arrhythmia that during long periods of sinus arrest, there is often failure of rescue escape beats to occur

Clinical findings
- The findings on auscultation are variable, from a markedly slow heart rate to a variable rhythm or with long pauses (associated with sinus arrest)
- The bradycardia-tachycardia syndrome sounds like periods of slow heart rate alternating with periods of a very fast heart rate
- There may be pulse deficits during the tachycardic episodes and no pulse produced during the periods of arrest

Persistent atrial standstill
- There is an absence of P waves
- The heart rate is usually slow
- QRS complexes are of a normal shape (sinoventricular escape rhythm)
- The atria are not seen to contract on fluoroscopy or echocardiography (atrial standstill)

Clinical findings
- The normal heart sounds will be heard (and associated pulse felt) in association with ventricular depolarisation
- The rate will vary in each case, although generally it is slower than normal (often less than 60/min)

Ventricular asystole
- Absence of any ventricular complexes and also usually any P waves
- This is cardiac arrest

Partial AV block
First degree AV block
- Delay in conduction through the AV node results in a prolonged PR interval – termed *first degree AV block*
- P wave and QRS complex are normal
- The P-R interval is prolonged (dog: >0.13 sec; cat: >0.09 sec)

Clinical findings
- No abnormality will be appreciated on auscultation or palpation of the pulse, and it cannot be distinguished from a normal sinus rhythm

Second degree AV block
- When the conduction occasionally fails to pass through the AV node it results in a P wave which is not followed by QRS-T complex – termed *second degree AV block*
- P wave is normal, but occasionally/ frequently (depending on severity) conduction fails to pass through the AV node resulting in the absence of a QRS complex

Clinical findings
- There will be occasional pauses in the rhythm associated with the absence of ventricular depolarisation
- On very careful auscultation the atrial contraction sounds ('A' sound or S4) can often be appreciated as a faint noise in association with atrial depolarisation

Complete (third degree) AV block
- Persistent failure of conduction to pass through the AV node
- A second pacemaker (at a lower rate than the SA node) discharges below the AV node to control the ventricles
- Slower pacemaker tissue in the ventricles may be from:
  - Lower AV node or bundle branches producing a normal QRS-T complex (junctional escape complexes) – approximately 60–70/min in the dog
  - Ventricular myocardial cells producing an abnormal QRS-T complex

(ventricular escape complexes) – approximately 30–40/min
- On the ECG, P-wave rate is faster than the QRS-T rate and they are independent of each other
- The P-P interval and the R-R interval are usually constant but with no relationship to each other

Note: Compare with AV dissociation (see p. 35).

Clinical findings
- A regular bradycardia is heard with, normally, a good palpable pulse (sometimes the escape rhythm is not regular).
- On very careful auscultation (sometimes using the bell of the stethoscope) the atrial contraction sounds (S4) can be faintly heard at a faster rate and not related to the normal lubb-dub of ventricular contraction.

Bundle branch blocks (intraventricular conduction defects)

The Bundle of His divides into left and right bundle branches, supplying the left and right ventricles respectively. The left bundle branch further divides into anterior and posterior fascicles. Block may occur in one or more of these conduction tissues, and in a number of combinations. The most commonly seen conduction defects seen in dogs and cats are:
- *Right bundle branch block (RBBB)*
- *Left bundle branch block (LBBB)*
- *Left anterior fascicular block (LAFB)*

These result in abnormal depolarisation patterns, as there will be a delay in depolarisation of the part of the ventricles supplied by the affected conduction tissue.
- The heart sounds and rhythm will sound normal with associated palpable pulses.

Right bundle branch block
- Failure/delay of impulse conduction through the RBB

- Depolarisation of the left ventricle occurs normally
- Depolarisation of the right ventricular mass occurs through the myocardial cell tissue resulting in a very prolonged complex (>0.07 sec)
- QRS complex has a deep (negative) S in leads I, II, III, aVF and is positive in aVR and aVL
- MEA is to the right
- Need to differentiate from a right ventricular enlargement pattern

Left bundle branch block
- Failure of conduction through the LBB
- Depolarisation of the right ventricle occurs normally
- Depolarisation of the left ventricle is delayed and occurs through the myocardial cell tissue resulting in a very prolonged complex (>0.07 sec)
- Positive complexes in leads I, II, III, aVF and negative in aVR and aVL
- Need to differentiate from a left ventricular enlargement pattern

Left anterior fascicular block
- Failure of conduction through the anterior fascicle of the LBB
- Results in a QRS duration that is usually normal
- Complexes have tall R waves in leads I and aVL and deep S waves (>R wave) in leads II, III and aVF
- MEA markedly to the left – approximately −60° in the cat

Ventricular pre-excitation
- This occurs when the depolarisation impulse bypasses the AV node through an accessory pathway, to stimulate the ventricle prematurely (pre-excite the ventricles)
- There are believed to be three possible accessory pathways in the dog
- On the ECG:

- ○ The P-R interval is very short
- ○ There may be a slur/notch (delta wave) in the upstroke of the R wave
- ○ The QRS may be slightly prolonged (as conduction is through the myocardial cells)
- ○ The rhythm is normal
- Pre-excitation may be associated with a paroxysmal supraventricular tachycardia (see later), occurring at a rate in excess of 300/min, by a re-entry mechanism, referred to as *Wolff-Parkinson-White (WPW) syndrome*

ABNORMALITIES DUE TO ECTOPIA

- Ectopic literally means in an abnormal place: when referring to the heart beat this means outside the SA node.
- Ectopic beats arise as a result of various mechanisms (e.g. re-entry, abnormal automaticity, after-depolarisations) due to a number of causes (e.g. electrolyte imbalances, hypoxia, cardiac pathology). The reader is referred to Chapter 7 and the references for more details.

Terminology
The electrocardiographic interpretation of arrhythmias due to ectopia requires an understanding of the terminology used. With terminology in place, interpretation becomes relatively easy.

The term *beat* implies that there has been an actual contraction. In 'ECG-speak' it is better to use the terms *complex* or *depolarisation* to describe waveforms on the electrocardiography.

Classification of ectopic complexes
Site of origin
- Ventricular
- Supraventricular

Timing
Ectopic complexes that occur before the next normal complex would have been due are termed *premature* and those that occur following a pause such as a period of sinus arrest or in complete heart block, are termed *escape* complexes.

Morphology
If all the ectopics in a tracing have a similar morphology to each other, they are referred to as *uniform*. Those in which there are different shapes as *multiform*.

Number of ectopics
Premature ectopic complexes may occur singly, in pairs or in runs of three or more – the latter is referred to as a *tachycardia*. A tachycardia may be continuous, termed *persistent* or *sustained*, or intermittent, termed *paroxysmal*.

Frequency
The number of premature ectopic complexes in a tracing may vary from occasional to very frequent. When there is a set ratio, such as one sinus complex to one ectopic complex it is termed *bigeminy*. One ectopic to two sinus complexes is termed *trigeminy*.

Ventricular premature complexes (VPCs)
- Arise from an ectopic focus/foci in the ventricles
- Depolarisation therefore occurs in a retrograde direction through the myocardial cells (not the conduction tissue)
- Thus the QRS complex is wide/prolonged and bizarre in shape, i.e. different from the QRS of a normal sinus complex
- It occurs prematurely, therefore a normal sinus depolarisation arriving at the AV node will meet ventricles which are refractory
- A P wave of a sinus complex will be hidden in the premature complex

- The AV node (and consequently the ventricles) will not be stimulated again until the next normal sinus depolarisation in the underlying rhythm – thus there will be an apparent pause (*compensatory pause*), and the normal rhythm is not disturbed, i.e. not *reset* (note that the depolarisation wave of a VPC cannot usually pass in a retrograde direction through the AV node to depolarise the atria)
- The T wave of a VPC is usually large and opposite in direction to the QRS
- As a general rule, VPCs that arise from the left ventricle have a negative QRS and those from the right ventricle a positive QRS
- A run of three or more VPCs is termed a *ventricular tachycardia* (VT)
- VT usually occurs at a rate in excess of 100/min

Clinical findings

- Occasional premature beats will sound like a 'tripping in the rhythm'. Depending upon how early the depolarisation occurs, the 'extra' premature beat may be heard or it might be silent, like a brief pause in the rhythm.
- There will be little or no pulse associated with the premature beat (i.e. there will be a pulse deficit).
- If the premature beats are more frequent, the tripping in the rhythm will start to make the heart rhythm sound more irregular.
- With very frequent premature beats, the heart rhythm can sound quite chaotic, and with a pulse deficit for each premature beat the pulse rate will be much slower than the heart rate.
- During a sustained ventricular tachycardia, however, the heart rhythm will sound fairly regular – pulses will probably be palpable, but reduced in strength, becoming weaker with faster heart rates.

Supraventricular premature complexes (SVPCs)

- Arise from an ectopic focus/foci above the ventricles, i.e. atria or AV node (junctional)
- Thus the ventricles are depolarised normally, producing a normal QRS complex
- The SVPC occurs prematurely
- Differentiating SVPCs into atrial premature complexes (APCs) or junctional premature complexes (JPCs) (see below) is difficult and of questionable clinical importance
- They need to be differentiated from wandering pacemaker, marked sinus arrhythmia and sinus tachycardia

Atrial premature complexes (APCs)

- An *atrial premature complex* (APC) arises in the atria, thus producing a P wave (referred to as a P′) that is abnormal in shape, being negative, positive or biphasic
- The P-R is usually prolonged
- The ectopic atrial depolarisation *resets* the SA node, such that the interval between the APC and the next sinus complex is the same as a normal R-R interval, i.e. there is *no compensatory pause* (sometimes referred to as having a *non-compensatory pause*)

Junctional premature complexes (JPCs)

- A *junctional premature complex* (JPC) arises within the AV node
- The depolarisation wave spreads through the ventricles and in a retrograde direction through the atria, thus producing a P′ wave that is abnormal in shape and usually negative in lead II
- The P′ wave may occur before, during or after the associated QRS complex
- If occurring before the QRS complex, the P′-R interval is usually shorter than normal
- The SA node is reset and there is no compensatory pause

Supraventricular tachycardia (SVT)

- A *supraventricular tachycardia* (SVT) is usually at a rate in excess of 160/min and fairly regular
- The P′ waves of a junctional tachycardia are usually negative in lead II and sometimes seen in the preceding T wave

Clinical findings

- Clinically it is not possible to distinguish ventricular premature beats from supraventricular premature beats.
- Occasional premature beats will sound like a 'tripping in the rhythm', with little or no pulse associated with the premature beat.

- If the premature beats are more frequent, the tripping in the rhythm will start to make the heart rhythm sound more irregular.
- With very frequent premature beats, the heart rhythm can sound quite chaotic, and, with a pulse deficit for each premature beat, the pulse rate will be much slower than the heart rate.
- During a sustained supraventricular tachycardia however, the heart rhythm will sound fairly regular – pulses will probably be palpable, but reduced in strength, becoming weaker with faster heart rates.

Escape Rhythms

When the dominant pacemaker (usually the SA node) fails to discharge for a long period, pacemaker tissue with a slower intrinsic rate (*junctional* or *ventricular*) may then discharge, i.e. the pacemaker tissue 'escapes' the control of the SA node. This is commonly seen in association with bradyarrhythmias (e.g. sinus bradycardia, sinus arrest, AV block). *Escape complexes* are sometimes referred to as *rescue beats*, because if they did not occur death would be imminent.

If no escape rhythm develops, i.e. there is no electrical activity of any kind, this is termed *asystole*. This is a terminal event unless electrical activity returns. If there is a failure of an escape rhythm during complete heart block, i.e. there are P waves but no QRS complexes, then this is termed *ventricular standstill*. Again, if ventricular electrical activity does not return death is imminent.

Junctional escapes are fairly normal in shape (i.e. junctional ectopic), whereas *ventricular* escapes are abnormal and bizarre (i.e. ventricular ectopic). A continuous junctional escape rhythm occurs at a rate of 60–70/min and a continuous ventricular escape rhythm occurs at a rate of <50/min. Either may be seen in complete AV block.

Since they are rescue beats they should not be suppressed. Treatment should be directed towards the underlying bradyarrhythmia.

AV dissociation

- *AV dissociation* refers to the situation in which the atria and ventricles are depolarised by separate independent foci
- Occurs due to:
  - Accelerated ventricular rhythm as a result of a junctional or ventricular focus or disturbed AV conduction
  - Depressed SA nodal function

- On the ECG:
  - Ventricular rate is faster than the atrial rate
  - P waves may occur before, during or after the QRS complex
  - P waves and QRS complexes are independent of each other
  - QRS complexes appear to 'catch up' on the P waves

- Compare to complete AV block (P wave rate greatly exceeds QRS rate)

Note: Complete AV block is one form of AV dissociation, but AV dissociation does not mean there is AV block.

Clinical findings

- The heart rhythm will sound fairly normal and the pulse should match the heart rate

Fibrillation and flutter

- Fibrillation means rapid irregular small movements of fibres and flutter means 'wave' or 'flap' quickly and irregularly
- Fibrillation and flutter occur by a mechanism termed *random re-entry*

Ventricular fibrillation (VF)

- This has nearly always a terminal effect, and causes cardiac arrest
- The depolarisation waves occur randomly throughout the ventricles
- There is therefore no significant co-ordinated contraction to produce any cardiac output
- If the heart is visualised, fine irregular movements of the ventricles may be seen, likened to a 'can of worms'
- The ECG shows *coarse* (larger) or *fine* (smaller), rapid, irregular and bizarre movements; no normal waves or complexes can be seen
- VF often follows ventricular tachycardia

Clinical findings

- No heart sounds are heard
- No pulse is palpable

Atrial fibrillation and flutter

- Depolarisation waves occur randomly throughout the atria
- On ECG
  - *Atrial flutter* is seen as rapid and regular, 'saw-toothed' type movements of the baseline, at a rate of 300–500/min. These are referred to as *F waves*. The QRS complex is normal and occurs at a more regular rate, often at a set frequency to the F waves.
  - *Atrial fibrillation* is recognised by the irregular chaotic ventricular (i.e. QRS) rate and rhythm (i.e. chaotic R-R intervals). The QRS complexes are not usually uniform due to variation in amplitude and in the majority of cases there are no recognisable P waves preceding the QRS complex. Sometimes fine irregular movements of the baseline are seen as a result of the atrial fibrillation waves, referred to as *f waves*, however these are frequently indistinguishable from baseline artifact (e.g. muscle tremor). The ventricular rate in dogs and cats is nearly always fast, as most cases are in congestive heart failure with a compensatory sympathetic drive (decreased AV node conduction time, reduced ventricular refractory period, thus increased rate).
- Atrial fibrillation is sometimes seen in giant breed dogs with no cardiac pathology – sometimes referred to as 'lone' AF. These dogs usually have a slower, more normal ventricular rate, as there is no increase in sympathetic drive because they are not in failure.

Clinical findings

- With AF the heart rhythm sounds chaotic (like 'slippers in a tumble dryer') and the pulse rate is often half the heart rate, especially with fast atrial fibrillation.
- This is a very common arrhythmia in dogs, and can be strongly suspected on auscultation when there is a chaotic rhythm and a 50% pulse deficit.
- Very frequent premature beats (ventricular or supraventricular) can mimic it.

OTHER ECG ABNORMALITIES

Low voltage QRS complexes

- QRS complexes will be smaller the further the electrodes are from the heart and depending upon the resistance to electrical conduction between the heart and the electrodes. For example, the ECG complexes are larger in precordial chest leads (because the electrodes are close to the heart).
- Complexes can be small in obese animals.
- Heavy filtering on the ECG machine can also reduce the amplitude of the ECG complexes significantly.

Causes of small QRS complexes

- Effusions (e.g. pericardial, pleural, ascitic)
- Hypothyroidism
- Pneumothorax

ECG features

An R wave amplitude less than 0.5 mV in the limb leads is considered small in dogs. QRS complexes are usually small in normal cats.

Electrical alternans

ECG features

This is an alternation in QRS amplitude that occurs nearly every other beat. It is most commonly seen with pericardial effusion.

Notching in the R wave

- Although these abnormalities can be seen commonly in heart disease in small animals, the significance of notches is debatable.
- Notches in the QRS complex are reported to occur with microscopic intramural myocardial infarction or associated with areas of myocardial fibrosis.

- Notches in the QRS complex are also seen with intraventricular conduction defects and a slight notch is sometimes also seen with ventricular pre-excitation in the upstroke of the R wave (delta wave).
- Notches can also be produced artifactually in tracings in which there is excessive muscle tremor or electrical interference.

S-T segment abnormalities

- S-T elevation is seen in:
  - Pericarditis
  - Severe ischaemia/infarction (e.g. full-wall thickness)
- S-T depression is seen in:
  - Endomyocardial ischaemia (e.g. cardio-myopathy, trauma)
  - Potassium imbalance
  - Digitalis toxicity

Abnormalities of the T wave

- The morphology of T waves in small animals is variable and the diagnostic value of T-wave changes is very limited compared to man. More value might be placed on T-wave changes compared to a previous recording in the same animal.
- The most common abnormal change is the development of large T waves. This can be associated with hyperkalaemia (see below) or myocardial hypoxia.

Hyperkalaemia

Hyperkalaemia is a well known cause of ECG abnormalities, but it must be remembered that a normal ECG would not exclude hyperkalaemia and serum electrolyte levels should always be measured (+/– an ACTH stimulation test performed) if this is suspected.

Causes

- Addison's disease
- Acute renal shutdown, e.g. feline urethral obstruction syndrome

- Diabetic ketoacidosis
- Severe skeletal muscle damage

ECG features

The ECG changes vary with increasing severity of the hyperkalaemia:

- There is a progressive bradycardia
- Increased amplitude of the T wave, appearing narrow and spiked
- Progressive decrease in amplitude of the R wave
- Progressive reduction in amplitude of the P wave
- Disappearance of the P wave, i.e. atrial standstill, with a sinoventricular rhythm
- Finally ventricular fibrillation or asystole

4 ECHOCARDIOGRAPHY

The aim of this text is to provide sufficient information for the practitioner to obtain a basic, but sound, introduction to echocardiography. Recommendations for how a beginner might approach echocardiography are provided below. The principles of ultrasound and detailed echocardiography are outwith the scope of this text and the interested reader should consult alternative sources.

- Cardiac ultrasound (echocardiography) consists of *two-dimensional* (2-D) and motion mode (*M-mode*) echocardiography and *Doppler ultrasound* (spectral and colour flow mapping).
- By combining the various aspects of echocardiography it is usually possible to diagnose cardiac disease accurately, detect abnormal blood flow (murmurs), quantify ventricular function and determine the severity of cardiac lesions in order to offer a prognosis.

EQUIPMENT

- Ultrasound system with real-time two-dimensional (2-D), M-mode, Doppler ultrasound and cardiac computer calculation packages.
- A sector scanning probe with a small transducer foot print is required to image between the rib spaces and allow good flexibility to obtain the various imaging planes. Ideally, a choice of transducers, from 3.5 MHz to 7.5 MHz, is necessary to image the range of sizes of dogs and cats. Two probes (e.g. 3.5 MHz and 7.5 MHz; or 5 MHz and 7.5 MHz) are required.
- An ability to store images so that the moving imaging can be reviewed frame by frame (scroll facility).
- To obtain good images of the heart, the animal is placed in lateral recumbency and scanned from the animal's dependent side. This brings the heart closer to the transducer and the weight of the heart presses the lungs to the side, reducing interference due to lung artifact. To achieve this position, it is necessary to lie the animal on a table with an appropriate U-shaped cut out (Figure 4.1).
- A record of the echocardiographic examination should be kept by video recording and/or by printer (or photography).

ANIMAL PREPARATION

- Clipping the animal's hair over the apex beat and down to the sternum is necessary.
- Wet skin with spirit or alcohol to reduce air artifact and apply acoustic ultrasound gel.
- The animal is restrained in lateral recumbency, on a suitable table. The

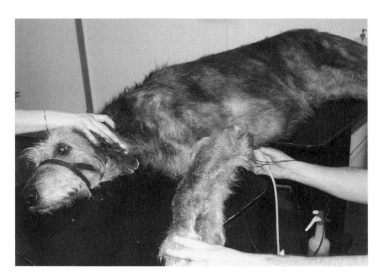

FIGURE 4.1   Photograph showing an Irish Wolfhound being scanned through a cut-out in a table.

underside foreleg should be pulled forward, thus removing the animal's elbow from the cardiac apex.

- Sedation is not usually required in dogs, but is sometimes necessary in cats to facilitate restraint. Sedation will not usually interfere with obtaining a diagnosis, but may alter assessment of severity, and therefore prognosis, of a cardiac disease.

- Cardiac ultrasound systems have a single-lead ECG monitor for the purposes of a timing reference. The clips should be attached and a good ECG trace noted prior to commencement.

TERMINOLOGY

- *Echolucent* (anechoic) – Does not reflect ultrasound and thus appears black, e.g. fluid
- *Echogenic* – Reflects ultrasound and shows tissue or tissue/fluid interface and appears white, e.g. heart walls and valves
- *Hypoechoic* – A relative term meaning one tissue reflects ultrasound less than another and thus appears darker, e.g. myocardium is hypoechic compared to valves
- *Hyperechoic* – A relative term that means one tissue reflects ultrasound more than another and thus appears whiter (brighter), e.g. endocardial fibrosis is hyperechoic compared to ventricular muscle

NORMAL ECHOCARDIOGRAPHIC EXAMINATION

- Appreciation of the abnormal, on echocardiography, does require familiarity with the normal in different breeds of dogs and in the cat. This can only be obtained by taking time to practice scanning in many normal animals.

- A good assessment of heart size and function can be made subjectively from 2-D images without taking measurements; in fact, incorrect measurements can lead the beginner to a misdiagnosis.

TWO-DIMENSIONAL (2-D) ECHOCARDIOGRAPHY

- Although it is possible to obtain an infinite number of 'slices' through the heart, there are a series of standard views.
- Despite the apparent complexity of echocardiography to the beginner there are a number of sequential steps recommended for a practitioner embarking on echocardiography (see below).
- The first two steps described below (right parasternal long and short axis views) will provide sufficient information to diagnose 80% of the cases seen in general practice competently.
- Once these two views can be competently achieved in the many different breeds of dog and in the cat, then progress to the other steps using appropriate texts (Boon 1998).

RECOMMENDATIONS FOR THE BEGINNER

Steps in learning echocardiography:
(1) Visualise the left atrium and ventricle from the right parasternal long axis view. Obtain left atrial diameter measurements made in 2-D
(2) Learn the short axis views from the right parasternal position. Obtain left ventricular chamber and atrial diameter measurements made in 2-D
(3) Scan the liver to assess degree of congestion from the size of the hepatic

veins and caudal vena cava (assessment of right heart failure)
(4) Obtain the other views from the right parasternal long axis
(5) Learn the use of M-mode and measurements made in M-mode. Routinely check all measurements obtained with M-mode, against those obtained in 2-D
(6) Visualise the various views from the left parasternal positions
(7) Learn the use of Doppler (spectral and colour)

STEP 1: Right parasternal long axis view of the left atrium and ventricle

- Hold the probe with your thumb on the notch/mark facing towards you.
- With the dog lying on its right side, begin by placing the transducer over the palpable apex beat on the dependent side (right 4th–6th intercostal space, just below the costochondral junctions) with the probe pointed vertically upwards, i.e. with no tilt, angulation or rotation.
- The heart should be found and then centred on the screen by moving the probe.
- With subtle tilting, angulation or rotation, a view of the left atrium, mitral valve and left ventricle should be obtained (Figure 4.2).
- This view should transect (in the third dimension) the middle of the left ventricle and atrium.
- The long axis of the heart is horizontal on the screen.
- The left ventricle is to the left side and the left atrium to the right side.
- The left ventricular chamber is slightly longer than it is wide, giving a 'bullet' shape to its chamber.
- The left atrium is fairly rounded in appearance.
- Measurement of left atrial diameter can

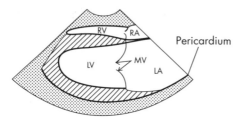

FIGURE 4.2 Diagrammatic representation of the right parasternal, long-axis view of the heart, showing the left atrium, left ventricle and mitral valve.

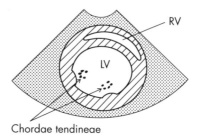

Chordae tendineae

FIGURE 4.4 Right parasternal, short-axis view at the level of the chordae tendineae.

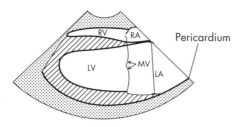

FIGURE 4.3 Diagram demonstrating measurement of maximal left atrial diameter in the long axis view (Rishniw & Erb 2000) (for normal values see Table 4.1, page 44).

be made from this view (Figure 4.3; Rishniw & Erb 2000).

- On the live image, the contractility of the left ventricle and movement of the mitral valve are observed.
- In the near field, the right ventricle and right atrium are seen, but the right heart is much smaller than the left heart, unless it is enlarged.
- The pericardium is not appreciated as a separate structure in normal animals, as it is in contact with the epicardium.

STEP 2: The short-axis views

- From the standard starting view described above (Figure 4.2), rotate the transducer anticlockwise 90° about

its axis (thumb rotates to the right, or caudally).

- This will result in a view which transects the left ventricle in its short axis, with the right ventricle surrounding the left ventricle from 11 o'clock to 4 o'clock.
- The transducer should be rotated or tilted to ensure that the left ventricle appears in true circular sections and is symmetrical. The sector beam can now be directed from the apex to the base of the heart by tilting the probe ventrally or dorsally at right angles to the plane of the sector beam.
- Tilt the probe until the *chordae tendineae* are seen arising from the papillary muscles (Figure 4.4). This is the level at which left ventricular measurements are made (see below on measurement of left ventricular chamber).
- Tilting the transducer further dorsally, the mitral valve begins to appear within the left ventricle. During diastole, the valves are open, and create an image often described as a 'fish-mouth'; in systole, when the valves close, the two cusps coapt to form an irregular line.
- Further dorsal tilting of the transducer will image a cross section of the aorta at valve level (Figure 4.5).

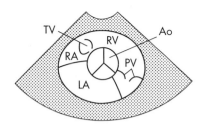

FIGURE 4.5 Echocardiogram showing the right parasternal, short axis view at the level of the aortic valve. The image created by the three cusps is sometimes described as a 'Mercedes Benz symbol' or an inverted 'Y'. To the lower left of the aorta (Ao) is the left atrium (LA) and below the aorta is the left auricle. The right side of the heart encircles the remaining portion of the aorta; the right atria (RA) and tricuspid valve (TV) to the upper left, the right ventricular (RV) outflow tract to the upper right and the pulmonary artery and its valve (PV) to the right.

Measurement of left ventricular chamber diameter from 2-D

- This is obtained from the short axis view at the level of the *chordae tendineae*. The tips of the mitral valve cusps are just apparent (Figure 4.4).
- Once that view is obtained, freeze the image, scroll back and check the quality of the images obtained.
- From a diastolic image (the left ventricular diameter is largest and coincides with the start of the QRS complex on the ECG) use the 2-D measuring facility to measure the inside of the left ventricle (LV), bisecting the LV between the *chordae tendineae* from endocardium of the septal wall to the endocardium on the free wall.
- Then find a systolic frame that follows (the LV diameter is smallest and is usually just after the T wave on the ECG). Again use the 2-D measuring facility to measure the LV diameter as above.

ASSESSMENT OF THE HEART ON 2-D ECHOCARDIOGRAPHY

The main objectives are to check for:
- Left or right atrial dilation
- Left or right ventricular chamber dilation or wall thickening (hypertrophy)
- Left ventricular wall motion
- Mitral valve thickening (endocardiosis)
- Ball thrombus or 'smoke' in a dilated left atrium in cats
- Pericardial effusion +/– right auricular or aortic-body tumour
- Pleural effusion
- Hepatic venous congestion

Left atrium
Left atrial size can be assessed by
- Subjective experience
- Comparison to the aorta and/or left ventricle
- By 2-D measurement from the long and short axis views (Figures 4.3 and 4.4).

Mitral valve
- The mitral valve cusps should be uniform in thickness, with no nodular thickening.
- Sometimes the attachment points of *chordae tendineae* to the cusp create slight echogenic reflections that can be mistaken for endocardiosis nodules.
- The mitral valve cusp should not cross a line between the annulus hinge point (not extend into the left atrium) – i.e. there should be no sign of cusp prolapse.
- The cusps should coapt during systole, with no gaps being seen.

Left ventricle
- Left ventricular size can be assessed by
  ○ Subjective experience
  ○ Measurements obtained by 2-D and M-mode from the short axis view at the level of the *chordae tendineae*

TABLE 4.1   Normal left atrial diameter for dogs obtained by 2-D measurement (long axis and short axis) as described by Rishniw & Erb (2000)

Weight (kg)	Left Atrium Long Axis Diameter Range (mm)	Left Atrium Short Axis Diameter Range (mm)
5	16–27	10–23
10	21–32	14–26
15	25–36	17–29
20	29–40	20–32
30	35–45	25–37
40	38–48	28–42
50	38–50	29–43
Ratio to aorta	<2:1	<1.6:1

- Measurement of left ventricular chamber diameter is one of the more important and useful measurements. The normal limits for each breed of dog do vary and it is best to compare results with that of normal for each breed, especially in dilated cardiomyopathy (DCM) (Table 4.2).
- For the beginner, measurement of left ventricular diameter is easiest to obtain from a 2-D image, provided the ultrasound machine has a scroll back facility. In due course, the ability to obtain satisfactory M-mode images will be acquired and measurements obtained by this modality. It is always recommended to obtain measurements by both methods, as a check for any errors.
- In short axis view the left ventricle should be round and symmetrical and the right ventricle seen as a slender crescent-shaped chamber surrounding half of the LV. The septal and LV free walls should be of a similar thickness. The papillary muscles should be similar and symmetrical.
- Left ventricular hypertrophy can be assessed subjectively and by measurement in 2-D and M-mode. Assessment of left ventricular septum and free-wall thickness is more important, in general practice, in cats when hypertrophic cardiomyopathy or systemic hypertension is suspected.
- Left ventricular contractility can be assessed subjectively and by measurement. The more useful measurements of LV *strength* are LV chamber systolic dimension, compared to normal for that breed (Table 4.2), and fractional shortening (FS).
- Calculation of the fractional shortening is obtained from the following equation:

Fractional shortening (FS) of the left

$$\text{ventricle} = \frac{\text{LVDd} - \text{LVDs}}{\text{LVDd}} \times 100 \ (\%)$$

(where LVDd is left ventricular chamber diameter in diastole, and LVDs is left ventricular chamber diameter in systole.)
- Fractional shortening (wall motion) is considered an estimate of contractility, but it varies with the preload and afterload on the heart and should not be overly relied upon.

TABLE 4.2   Published normal left ventricular internal diameter measurements and fractional shortening published for individual breeds of dog

Breed	Parameter	LVDd (mm)	LVDs (mm)	FS (%)	Reference
Irish Wolfhound	Mean (SD)	53.2 (4.0)	35.4 (2.8)	34 (4.5)	Vollmar (1999a)
Irish Wolfhound	Mean (SD)				Brownlie & Cobb
	Male	53.3 (4.5)	38.6 (3.7)	28.2 (4.3)	(1999)
	Female	51.8 (4.0)	36.9 (4.2)	29.1 (4.3)	
Spanish Mastiff	Mean (SD)	47 (1.4)	29 (1.1)	39 (1.6)	Bayon et al. (1994)
Great Dane	Range	44–59	34–45	18–36	Koch et al. (1996)
Deerhound	Mean (SD)	51 (5)	34 (5)	33 (6)	Vollmar (1998)
Newfoundland	Mean (SD)	45.3 (3.8)	33.7 (2.9)	25 (2.9)	Dukes-McEwan (1999)
Saluki	Mean (SD)	45 (4)	33 (4)	28	Brownlie (1999)
Greyhound	Range	40–49	29–38	17–35	Page et al. (1993)
English Pointer	Mean (SD)	39.2 (2.4)	25.3 (2.4)	35.5 (4.0)	Sisson & Schaeffer (1991)
Golden Retriever	Range	37–51	18–35	27–55	Morrison et al. (1992)
Dobermann	Normal range	32.7–45.2	25.7–37.9	13–30	O'Grady & Horne (1995)
Afghan	Range	33–52	20–37	24–48	Morrison et al. (1992)
Boxer	Range	40 (4.5)	27 (4.0)	32 (7)	Herrtage (1994)
Cocker Spaniel	Mean (SD)	33.8 (3.3)	22.2 (2.8)	34.3 (4.5)	Gooding et al. (1986)
Corgi	Range	28–40	12–23	33–57	Morrison et al. (1992)
Cavalier King Charles Spaniel	Mean (SD)	29 (3)	20 (2.5)	33 (4.5)	Häggström et al. (2000)
Beagle	Range	18–33	8–27	20–70	Crippa (1992)
Miniature Poodle	Range	16–28	8–16	35–57	Morrison et al. (1992)

- Left or right ventricular hypertrophy will be appreciated with moderate to severe congenital defects causing an outflow obstruction such as aortic and pulmonic stenosis.

Right heart

- The right heart is usually assessed subjectively, but as a guideline the right ventricular chamber is approximately one third the size of the left ventricle.

TABLE 4.3 Normal left ventricular, left atrial and aortic diameter values for cats (Bonagura *et al.* 1985)

Normal Left Ventricular Values	(mm)
LVd	11.0–16.0
LVs	6.0–10.0
IVSd	2.5–5.0
IVSs	5.0–9.0
LVPWd	2.5–5.0
LVPWs	4.0–9.0
LA	8.5–12.5
Ao	6.5–11.0
FS%	29–55%

- The right atrium is smaller than the left atrium.
- The interventricular and interatrial septa should both be fairly straight. Bowing towards one side would suggest volume/pressure load in the opposite chamber.
- Occasionally the high membranous ventricular septum or the atrial septum (where they are particularly thin) are not clearly seen, thus mimicking a septal defect – this is referred to as echo drop-out.
- The tricuspid valve annulus is a little closer to the ventricular apex than the mitral valve.
- Examination for right-sided congestive failure can be assisted by ultrasound examination of the liver for enlargement/congestion and the hepatic veins for enlargement.

Fluid
- Pericardial fluid can be seen as an echolucent area surrounding the heart but contained within the echogenic pericardium.
- Pleural fluid can be seen as an echolucent fluid surrounding the heart/pericardium.

M-MODE ECHOCARDIOGRAPHY

- Motion-mode (M-mode) echocardiography is obtained by placing the cursor line through the heart, in an area of interest, and displaying the movement of the heart against time through that single line (time-motion graph/display). Time is on the X axis and motion on the Y axis. The ECG provides a timing reference.
- M-mode echocardiography is generally used when performing measurements or observing the motion of structures over time.

DOPPLER ECHOCARDIOGRAPHY

- In Doppler echocardiography, ultrasound is transmitted towards the area of interest in the heart, and when it is reflected by a moving structure, e.g. red blood cells, the reflected ultrasound has a change in frequency which can be used to calculate the direction of movement and speed of the red blood cells.
- There are different forms of Doppler ultrasound used in echocardiography:
  ○ Spectral Doppler
  ○ Continuous wave (CW) Doppler
  ○ Pulsed Doppler
    – low pulsed repetition frequency (LPRF)
    – high pulsed repetition frequency (HPRF)
  ○ Colour-flow mapping
- To record blood-flow velocities, the Doppler beam or sample volume must be in line (parallel) with the direction of flow, and not exceeding 20° out of line in three dimensions.
- Mild regurgitation from the pulmonic valve has been found to occur in up to 70% of normal dogs.

Note: Normal pulmonary artery to right ventricular pressures will result in a regurgitant jet velocity of approximately 2.2 m/s.

- Regurgitation from the tricuspid valve occurs in 50% of normal dogs.

Note: Normal right ventricular to right atrial pressures will result in a regurgitant jet velocity of approximately 2.8 m/s.

- Mild regurgitation from the aortic or mitral valves has been found in 10–15% of normal dogs.
- Blood flow within the heart is usually laminar and the Doppler velocity display (termed the *spectral velocity display*) will show that the majority of red cells accelerate together to a similar peak velocity and decelerate at a similar rate. This gives a spectral velocity display that is referred to as a *clean envelope* or described as having minimal *spectral dispersion*.
- Abnormal or turbulent flow, such as occurs distal to an obstruction, will produce a spectral velocity display that has widespread spectral dispersion.
- Abnormalities in blood flow (*disturbed flow*) may be due to valvular regurgitation, stenosis or cardiac shunts.
- The pressure gradient between any two chambers, or the ventricles and great vessels, can be estimated from the peak velocity of blood flow between the two. For example, if the velocity is within the normal range proximal to a stenosis and grossly elevated distal to it, the pressure gradient that is required to produce the peak velocity can be estimated from the modified Bernoulli equation:

pressure gradient $= 4(V_2^2 - V_1^2)$

(where V_2 is the peak velocity distal to the obstruction and V_1 is the peak velocity proximal to the obstruction)

CONTRAST ECHOCARDIOGRAPHY

This is a useful and easy technique that is used to check for reverse shunting defects.

- Injection of a suspension of microbubbles into a peripheral vein, observing the 2-D image for the presence of shunts.
- The microbubbles can be created by pushing intravenous fluid (e.g. Haemaccel) rapidly to-and-fro between two syringes connected by a three way tap. When a suspension of bubbles has been produced, the three way tap is opened to a previously-placed intravenous cannula and the fluid injected. Only a small amount of fluid is required, e.g. 1–2 ml for a medium-sized dog.
- This technique requires an assistant to perform the injection, while the echocardiographer maintains adequate visualisation of the area of interest. It is recommended that the procedure is recorded on video, so that repeat viewings of the injection may be studied.
- The microbubbles are quickly seen to cause the right atrium, ventricle and pulmonary artery to become opaque.
- The presence of right-to-left shunts can be seen as the microbubbles pass into the left side of the heart.
- If there is a reverse shunting patent ductus arteriosus, bubbles will not be seen in the left heart, but will cross into the aorta through the ductus and can then be seen by scanning the abdominal aorta.

ECHOCARDIOGRAPHIC FEATURES OF THE COMMON HEART DISEASES

MITRAL VALVE DISEASE

- The left atrium is dilated
- The diameter of the atrium usually exceeds the diameter of the ventricle
- Left ventricular wall motion (contractility) is normally good
- The left ventricle can often also appear dilated
- The mitral valve cusps may appear nodular – although this can be difficult to appreciate in mild cases
- The tips of the cusps may not meet at the point of closure during systole
- The mitral valve cusps may be seen to bow/parachute/prolapse into the left atrium
- If the tricuspid valve is also affected, the right heart may be dilated

DILATED CARDIOMYOPATHY

- The left ventricle appears dilated and rounded (globoid)
- The wall motion (contractility) of the ventricle is reduced
- The ventricular walls may also appear thinner than normal

- The left atrium is usually dilated, but no more so than the left ventricle
- The right heart may also appear dilated

HYPERTROPHIC CARDIOMYOPATHY IN CATS

- The left ventricular wall and papillary muscles appear thickened
- Contractility is normal
- The left atrium may or may not be dilated

PERICARDIAL EFFUSION

- The pericardial sac is filled with effusion – a large, echolucent, filled space surrounding the heart
- A pericardial echodensity can usually be appreciated around the outside edge of this space
- The right heart often seems small
- The walls of the right atrium and ventricle may be seen to collapse at times
- The left heart usually appears normal

5 FURTHER INVESTIGATIVE TECHNIQUES

CLINICAL PATHOLOGY

HAEMATOLOGY AND BIOCHEMISTRY PROFILES

Routine haematology and biochemistry profiles are rarely of use in the diagnosis of cardiorespiratory diseases, but will give valuable information about the health status of the patient in general. It can show, for example, if the disease of the cardiac or respiratory systems is causing secondary problems with other body systems or if diseases of other body systems are present that might mimic the clinical signs of cardiac and respiratory diseases.

Haematology
- Identification of haematological diseases such as anaemia or polycythaemia
  - Anaemia (<20%) may produce a haemic cardiac murmur
- Checking for clotting defects
  - Primary
  - Secondary (e.g. angiostrongylosis)
- Circulating neutrophilia in bacterial bronchopneumonia
- Circulating eosinophilia in parasitism or pulmonary infiltrate with eosinophilia (PIE)

Biochemistry profiles
- Identification of systemic illness
- Identification of suspected endocrinopathies
- Identification of secondary effects on hepatic and renal function
- Hepatopathy due to hepatic venous congestion

- Alanine aminotransferase (ALT) and serum alkaline phosphatase (SAP or ALP) are often mildly elevated with hepatic congestion
- Pre-renal azotaemia due to congestive heart failure or dehydration (e.g. over-diuresis)
  - Urea elevated proportionally much more so than creatinine or phosphorus
- Electrolyte disturbances
  - Depletion may be seen with aggressive diuresis
  - Na^+, K^+, Ca^{++}, Mg^{++}
- Identify changes that could impair drug distribution, metabolism and excretion, such as hypokalaemia
- Biochemical indicators of myocardial damage
  - Lactate dehydrogenase, fractions 1 and 2
    - Used in man, rarely in animals
  - Cardiac troponin-I (cTnI) – normal <0.3 ng/ml
    - Marker of cardiac myocyte injury
    - This is a useful parameter
    - Markedly elevated with diseases such a myocarditis or ischaemia
    - Often elevated with feline cardiomyopathies
    - Mildly elevated with many other heart diseases
- Biochemical indicators of myocardial failure
  - Natriuretic peptides are becoming increasingly available
    - Useful markers that help to recognise the presence of cardiomegaly/congestive heart failure

- Particularly useful in differentiating cardiac from respiratory disease
○ Atrial natriuretic peptide (proANP)
  - Released from atrial myocardial cells when stretched/dilated
  - ProANP <1350 fmol/l is normal, i.e. heart failure or enlargement are most unlikely
  - ProANP > 1750 fmol/l – heart failure very likely
○ Brain (ventricular) naturetic peptide (BNP)
  - Assay under development for animals

Dynamic biochemistry profiles

Dynamic biochemistry profiles can supply confirmation of suspected endocrinopathies.

SEROLOGY TESTS

- Serology can be used to assess possible infection or possible exposure to a variety of agents, including *Aspergillus fumigatus* (although false positive and false negative results do occur) and other fungi, *Toxoplasma gondii* and other protozoal agents and viral infections.
- Virus isolation is usually required to confirm respiratory viral infections, such as with feline herpes virus (FHV) or calici virus (FCV).

BLOOD GAS ANALYSIS

Blood gas analysis is of great benefit in assessing respiratory function and is superior to all other tests in determining the degree of respiratory impairment. Blood gas analysis is used to monitor arterial carbon dioxide and oxygen partial pressures, and provides information on the severity of hypoxaemia, the degree of ventilation–perfusion mismatch and hypoventilation, the need for oxygen supplementation and the progression of disease. Monitoring of venous gas partial pressures is not as useful and can be difficult to interpret.

PROCEDURE

- Arterial sampling
- Use a heparinised syringe
- The femoral artery is most commonly used
- Restraint is needed to allow access
- Place in lateral recumbency with the upper leg retracted
- Palpate the femoral artery in the inguinal region
- Direct needle at right angles to the vessel

- If in the artery the syringe should fill easily
- Withdraw the needle and apply digital pressure for five minutes
- Immediately mix the blood in the syringe, expel air bubbles and cap
- Preferably analyse immediately, or place in ice-water (not just ice) and analyse within six hours
- Correction for the patient's body temperature performed by the automatic analyser

Sampling can be stressful and, in the respiratory compromised patient, the benefits of arterial sampling may not necessarily out-weigh the risks. Arterial sampling can be difficult and will need practice before competence is achieved. The less sampling an operator is undertaking the less likely they will be successful.

INTERPRETATION

Hypoxia

- Normal mean arterial oxygen tension is 95 mmHg in the dog and 105 mmHg in the cat

- Hypoxia can be defined as a PaO_2 of 80 mmHg or less and oxygen supplementation is recommended if PaO_2 falls below 60 mmHg

Causes
- Inadequate oxygen delivery
  - Anaesthesia
  - Inappropriate anaesthetic settings or anaesthetic equipment faults
  - Poorly ventilated environment
- Ventilation–perfusion mismatch
  - Lower airway and lung parenchymal diseases
  - Pulmonary thromboembolism
- Hypoventilation
  - Upper airway obstruction
  - Pleural effusion
  - CNS depression
  - Neuromuscular disease
- Diffusion abnormalties
  - Very few specific entities identifiable in dogs and cats
  - Consequence of advanced lung parenchymal disease

Hypercapnia
- Normal arterial carbon dioxide tension is 37 mmHg in dogs and 31 mmHg in cats
- Hypercapnia can be defined as $PaCO_2$ above 43 mmHg in the dog and 36 mmHg in the cat
  - Respiratory acidosis due to hypoventilation
  - Upper airway obstruction
  - Neuromuscular disease
  - Pleural effusion
  - Thoracic cage diseases
- Hypocapnia can be defined as $PaCO_2$ less than 32 mmHg in the dog and 26 mmHg in the cat
  - Respiratory alkalosis due to hyperventilation
  - Fever, excitement, pain, stress
  - Pulmonary thromboembolism (due to hyperventilation)

Alveolar–arterial PO_2 gradient ([A – a]PO_2)
- The A – a gradient is the difference between the measured pressure of oxygen in the blood stream (a) and the calculated pressure of oxygen in the alveolar sacs (A)
- The higher the gradient the more problem there is in oxygen reaching the blood
- The A – a gradient helps to determine if the measured PaO_2 is acceptable or if there is lung disease
- Formulae for calculation of the A – a gradient:

$$PAO_2 = 150 - (PaCO_2 \times 1.1)$$
$$P[A - a]O_2 = PAO_2 - PaO_2$$

- Identification of cause of hypoxia
  - Hypoventilation
    – Hypoxia with hypercapnia
  - Ventilation–perfusion mismatch
    – Hypoxic with normocapnia (or hypocapnia)
- A – a gradient
  - Normal probably less than 10 mmHg (exact figure not known)
  - Ventilation–perfusion mismatch more than 20 mmHg
  - The greater the gradient, the greater the venous admixture (V/Q mismatch)
  - Hypoventilation less than 15 mmHg

ACID–BASE STATUS

Interpretation is conventionally made without correction for body temperature. It is satisfactory to assess acid–base status from either an arterial or venous blood sample.
- Base excess and HCO_3 represent the amount of alkali
- Base excess is considered a more independent, and therefore more useful, measurement of alkali
- CO_2 is acidic and therefore a measure of the amount of acid

- pH homeostasis is primarily dependent upon the balance between CO_2 and HCO_3

Interpretation

Step 1 Check pH (Table 5.1)
- If pH is within the normal range, but either base excess or CO_2 are abnormal, then there is a derangement but compensation has occurred (or there has been a complicated mixed acid–base derangement)

Step 2 Check base excess (or HCO_3) in relation to pH
- An increase in base excess (excess alkali) raises the pH, and a low base excess lowers the pH
- If the base excess is shifted in the same direction as the pH, then base excess is the culprit, i.e. primary metabolic disorder (Table 5.2)

TABLE 5.1 Abnormalities as indicated by pH

pH Value	Abnormality
<7.4	Acidosis
>7.4	Alkalosis
<7.36	Acidaemia
>7.44	Alkalaemia

TABLE 5.2 Interpretation of base excess in relation to pH, where base excess is shifted in the same direction as pH

pH	Base Excess	Interpretation
High	High	Metabolic alkalosis
Low	Low	Metabolic acidosis

TABLE 5.3 Interpretation of base excess in relation to pH, where base excess is shifted in the opposite direction as pH

pH	Base Excess	Interpretation
High	Normal or low	Likely respiratory alkalosis, check CO_2
Low	Normal or high	Likely respiratory acidosis, check CO_2

- If the pH is high, but the base excess normal or low (no excess in alkali), then base excess cannot be the cause of the high pH
- If the pH is low but the base excess is normal or high, then base excess cannot be the cause of the low pH (Table 5.3)

Step 3 Check CO_2
- A high CO_2 will lower the pH (and vice versa)
- If the CO_2 is shifted in the opposite direction of the pH, then CO_2 is the culprit, i.e. primary respiratory disorder
- If both base excess and CO_2 are shifted in a direction that would contribute to an abnormal pH then a mixed metabolic and respiratory abnormality exists

Step 4 Is there compensation?
- Once the primary disturbance has been established, check the other value (i.e. base excess or CO_2)
- If the other value is abnormal and in a direction that should push the pH in the opposite direction to the primary disturbance, then compensation is occurring
- Respiratory compensation is fast and is complete within 12–24 hours
- Metabolic compensation is slow and is complete within 2–5 days

CAUSES OF ACID–BASE DISTURBANCES

Metabolic acidosis

Due to an acid load:
- Accumulation of lactate (lactic acidosis)
- Untreated diabetes (diabetic ketoacidosis)
- Ingestion of methanol, alcohol or ethylene glycol
- Failure of kidneys to excrete acids
- Loss of HCO_3 – e.g. diarrhoea, renal tubular disease

Metabolic alkalosis

- Vomiting of acidic stomach contents
- Hypokalaemia
- Renal loss, e.g. diuresis

Respiratory acidosis

CO_2 accumulation – inadequate alveolar ventilation:
- Upper airway obstruction
- Lower airway obstruction, e.g. asthma
- Impaired alveolar filling, e.g. bronchopneumonia
- Respiratory depression by drugs

Respiratory alkalosis

- Occurs due to hyperventilation, e.g. psychological, respiratory stimulants, anaesthetic over-ventilation
- Reduction in oxygen, e.g. anaemia, pulmonary disease, septicaemia, pulmonary oedema, high altitude

AIRWAY ENDOSCOPY

Airway endoscopy is very important in the diagnosis of respiratory diseases. It allows the direct visualisation of the respiratory tract and assists in the accurate sampling of material for cytological analysis.

RHINOSCOPY

Applications
- Visualisation of the nasal passages
- Retrieval of foreign bodies
- Improved sampling

Equipment
- Otoscope
  - Visualisation of rostral part of the nasal cavities
- Dental mirror and retractors
  - Visualisation of caudal nasal cavities
- Rigid arthroscope
  - Good visualisation
  - Flushing or biopsy capability

- Easily traumatise mucosa causing bleeding
- Flexible fibre-optic endoscope
  - Very good visualisation
  - More manoeuvrable and versatile compared to rigid scopes
  - Less traumatic than rigid endoscopes
  - Visualisation of caudal nasal passages Retroflex technique can be used
    Main limiting factor is external diameter of the scope

Procedure

Rhinoscopy is undertaken as part of a series of investigative techniques and not on its own or in isolation from other diagnostic tests. Investigation of nasal cases should be planned and carried out in a logical and complete fashion. It is time-consuming and expensive.
- General anaesthesia required
- Pre-anaesthetic and pre-rhinoscopy blood work-up
  - Significant haemorrhage a possibility

○ Coagulation profiles, buccal mucosal bleeding time, platelet count
- Reduce possibility of aspiration of fluids and blood
  ○ Cuffed endotracheal tube placed
  ○ Pack oropharynx with swabs
- Carry out radiography etc. prior to rhinoscopy
- Inspect the oral cavity first
  ○ Dental disease
  ○ Oronasal fistulas
  ○ Palate defects

Entry to rostral nasal cavities

- This can be difficult
- Pass the scope ventromedially at the entrance to the external nares
- Straighten the scope and advance into the common meatus
- Flushing with saline through the scope can assist in passage and visualisation
- Nasal conchae seen in the lateral position
- Nasal meatus seen directly in front

Entry to the caudal nasal passages

- Place biopsy catheter in the biopsy channel
- Retroflex the tip of the endoscope and pass beyond the caudal border of the soft palate
- Draw the endoscope rostrally
- The caudal choanae and nasopharynx can be visualised
- Advance the biopsy catheter and sample
- Avoid keeping the scope tip in this over-flexed position for prolonged periods

Findings and interpretation

Normal findings
- Rostral nasal cavities
  ○ Limited view due to the cavity being filled with the ethmo- and maxillo-turbinates
  ○ Pink nasal mucosa with visible vessels
  ○ Some secretions
- Caudal nasal cavities

○ Wide open structure
○ Smooth, pink mucosa with clearly visible vessels
○ Minimal secretions

Abnormal findings

- Rostral nasal cavities
  ○ Turbinate destruction
  ○ More open nasal cavity
  ○ Mucosal hyperaemia, erosions, adherent material
  ○ Mucosal hypertrophy
  ○ Mucopurulent secretions, blood, fungal plaques
  ○ Masses
  ○ Foreign bodies
- Caudal nasal cavities
  ○ Mucosal hyperaemia
  ○ Mucopurulent secretions
  ○ Masses
  ○ Foreign bodies
  ○ Nasal mites (in enzootic areas)

Note: It is easy to cause haemorrhage, even in normal nasal passages.

LARYNGOSCOPY

Applications

- Examination of the oropharyngeal and laryngeal areas
- Assessment of laryngeal function

Equipment

- Sophisticated equipment is not required
- Penlight, with probe to move structures out of view
- Laryngoscope

Procedure

- Carry out inspection under general anaesthesia
- Place in sternal recumbency
- Hold mouth open, with tongue pulled forward over lower incisor teeth
- Use a probe to move soft palate or epiglottis out of the line of view

- Inspect soft tissues of the oropharynx including the tonsils
- Assess the length of the soft palate
- Assess size of glottic opening
- Identify normal laryngeal movement during inspiration
  - Inspect under very light general anaesthesia, such that gag reflex is present and jaw tone strong
  - Doxapram (Dopram-V) at 0.5–1.0 mg/kg i/v – induces hyperpnoea making laryngeal assessment easier
  - Check arytenoids are *actively abducting on inspiration* and not just moving passively with breathing
  - Secondary features are inflammation and/or erosion of the mucosal surface of the arytenoids and sometimes the presence of saliva in the pharynx or even within the trachea
- Inspect aryepiglottic folds and the epiglottis
- Identify and inspect the vocal folds and laryngeal saccules

Findings and interpretation
Normal findings
- Mucosa appears pink and there are minimal secretions
- Structures are readily identified
- There is no tissue redundancy
- Soft palate extends to the caudal pole of the tonsils
- Glottis opens during inspiration (under light anaesthesia)
- Vocal cords are thin and the laryngeal saccules not readily visible

Abnormal findings
- The mucosa looks hyperaemic
- There are excessive secretions
- Lymphoid nodules are visible on mucosal surfaces
- The soft palate is excessively long
- Redundancy of soft tissues occluding the oropharynx

- Failure to abduct the arytenoids during inspiration (narrowing of *rima glottides*)
- Laryngeal oedema
- Thickened vocal cords
- Eversion of the laryngeal saccules

BRONCHOSCOPY

Applications
- Inspection of the airways
  - Mucosal alterations
  - Occlusion of airways
  - Identify secretions
- Improve accuracy of sampling
- Endoscopic retrieval of airway foreign bodies

Equipment
- Rigid endoscope
  - Rarely used nowadays
- Flexible fibre-optic endoscope (bronchoscope)
  - Most widely used
  - Lengths above 80 cm are most suitable
  - Suitable diameters for small animal work (<9 mm)
  - Wide price range
- Video-endoscope (usually gastroscopes)
  - Longer working length
  - Suitable for large dogs
  - Limited diameters available
  - Expensive

There are reasonably priced veterinary flexible fibre-optic endoscopes available. They have a longer working length than human bronchoscopes, but the image tends to be of lesser quality. The smaller the scope diameter, the poorer the quality of the image.

Procedure
- Review thoracic radiographs to get information on likely localisation of disease

- General anaesthesia required, with competent anaesthetic monitoring
- Sternal or lateral recumbency acceptable, but sternal reduces chances of positional atelectasis of dependent lung lobes
- Intubate and supply supplemental oxygen/anaesthetic gases
- Extubate if the trachea needs inspection (suspected tracheal collapse)
- Rapid initial inspection
  - Reduce risk of prolonged airway occlusion
  - Reduce airway reaction (mucus secretion) to the endoscope
  - Give guidance as to what areas might need most time for inspection
- Inspect *trachea*
  - Colour of mucosa
  - Presence of secretions
  - Collapse
- Inspect *carina*
  - As for trachea
  - Appearance of entrance to mainstem bronchi
  - Presence of nodules
- *Mainstem bronchi*
  - As for trachea
  - Check for occlusion or dynamic collapse during the respiratory cycle
- Inspect *lobar bronchi* in following order:
  - Right cranial, right middle, right accessory, right caudal, left cranial (including cranial and caudal divisions) and left caudal
- For each lobar bronchus check for the following
  - Excessive secretions

- Mucosal changes (hyperaemia, pallor, patchy surface, erosive lesions, nodular changes)
- Blood or blood-tinged secretions
- Dynamic airway collapse

Findings and interpretation
Normal findings
- Mucosa has a light pink colour
- Mucosa has a slightly glistening appearance
- Blood vessels are visible beneath epithelium
- Tracheal cartilage rings clearly visible
- No secretions, or very little, visible in any airways

Abnormal findings
- Mucosal changes
  - Hyperaemic mucosa
  - Mucosal erosions
  - Pale mucosa
  - Nodular changes on mucosal surface
  - Sub-epithelial vessels difficult to see
- Increased secretions
  - Generalised or localised (lobar)
  - Clear mucus
    - Mucus secretion is often induced by the presence of the endoscope
  - Mucopurulent material
  - Blood-tinged material
- Tracheal collapse
- Collapse of carina and/or mainstem bronchi
- Dynamic collapse of lobar bronchi
- Bronchiectasis (pathological dilatation)
- Airway foreign bodies
- Mural masses (very rare)

AIRWAY AND LUNG SAMPLING

Obtaining material from the respiratory system for cytology, culture or histopathology is crucial in the investigation of respiratory disease, as it is more likely to give a definitive diagnosis than any other diagnostic test. Biopsy sampling tends to be technically difficult, invasive and may have unacceptable levels of morbidity, but obtaining material for cytology and culture is readily achievable.

Brush biopsy techniques can also be used to get representative cytology samples from the nasal passages and the trachea and bronchi.

CYTOLOGY SAMPLING

Nasal wash

- Nasal flushing with a urinary catheter or Foley catheter
- Requires anaesthesia
- Good return
- Problems of contamination

Transtracheal wash

- Catheter passed via 14G needle inserted through the cricothyroid ligament
- Carried out conscious or under heavy sedation
- Variable return

Tracheobronchial sampling

- Blind sampling
  - Catheter passed *per os* (preferably via endotracheal tube)
  - Reasonable return, but might get no return
  - Only usually sample trachea or main-stem bronchi
- Endoscope guided
  - Catheter directed to area of interest
  - Accurate sampling of material possible
  - Good return

Bronchoalveolar lavage (BAL) sampling

- See boxed text below for technique
- Requires endoscopic guidance
- Only method of guaranteeing material from distal airways and alveoli
- Very good return

Technique for BAL Sampling

- Load five or six 20 ml syringes with warm (non-bacteriostatic) saline. Suitable volumes are approximately 0.5 ml/kg per syringe (usually to a maximum of 20 ml).
- Pass the flexible endoscope into the selected bronchus almost occluding it, then advance the endoscopic catheter (but remaining within view).
- Flush the catheter with one syringeful of saline and aspirate *immediately*. Watch that the catheter is not occluded by the side wall of the bronchus. The catheter often needs to be moved back and forth to prevent this.
- Repeat this with 4–6 flushes, until a suitable sample is retrieved. Two flushes might be sufficient.
- Up to 50% of the sample volume can often be retrieved, with the remainder being absorbed by the lung.
- Foaming of the sample indicates the presence of surfactant from the alveoli, and is therefore an indication of a 'good' lavage.
- A useful sample will usually contain discharge from the airway (mucoid or purulent) and will have a cloudy appearance.

Sample Handling

- Preparation of top-quality smears is vital for cell preservation – this must be done as soon as possible (within 30 minutes).
- Pool the collected material and divide into two aliquots and centrifuge.
- Decant the supernatant (saline) with a pipette leaving the sediment and a small volume of saline in the pot.

- Mix the saline and sediment by drawing the sample in and out of the pipette until a uniform homogenous sample is obtained.
- Place a spot of the BAL fluid sample onto a number of glass slides, use the squash and pull apart method to spread the sample and *air dry rapidly* with a hairdryer on a cold setting (this is vital for cell preservation).
- Submit samples to an experienced cytologist – it is important to communicate with your cytologist on the quality of the samples you submitted.
- In the other aliquot, dip a swab (with transport medium) into the spot of sediment and submit for culture and sensitivity.

Interpretation of the cytologist's report

Accurate assessment of the primary airway cell response is the key to diagnosing many lower airway diseases, but there are pitfalls in obtaining good samples and upper airway contamination can cause confusion.

- A good BAL sample should be cellular, with the presence of macrophages indicating the lavage has reached alveolar level. An excessive amount of epithelial cells would indicate upper airway contamination. The presence of squamous cells or *Simonsiella* would indicate oral contamination.

Note: This is important when interpreting any culture result.

- The presence of red blood cells suggests bleeding into the airways, which may be due to the sampling procedure, FBs or neoplasia (the cytologist can differentiate between fresh or chronic haemorrhage).
- A significant growth on culture should, but not necessarily, be associated with intracellular bacteria and absence of contamination in the cytology report.

NORMAL BAL CYTOLOGY

Small cell numbers
- Macrophages – 60–80%
- Neutrophils 1–20%

- Eosinophils 5–20%
- Lymphocytes 1–10%

Note: A good BAL sample should demonstrate the presence of macrophages

Abnormal airway cytology
- Increased cell numbers
  - Neutrophils and macrophages (non-specific inflammation)
  - Neutrophil and/or macrophage morphological changes
    - Evidence of cell degeneration
    - Evidence of cell differentiation
    - Intracellular bacteria
  - Eosinophils – allergic, feline asthma syndrome or parasitic disease
  - Neoplastic cells
- Increased quantities of mucus

SAMPLING FOR CULTURE

- Bacteriology results are usually only significant when a significant number of bacteria are found on cytology
- False positive results are not uncommon, due to culture of normal flora
- Same techniques as for cytology sampling. If collecting a wash take an aliquot of the collected material and process for culture (proper transport media: bacterial, fungal, viral)
- Nasal swab
  - Guarded swab to reduce risk of contamination

BIOPSY SAMPLING

- Nasal biopsy
  - Blind biopsy
    - Grabbing or biting forceps
  - Rhinotomy biopsy
    - Rhinotomy surgical pack required
- Airway biopsy
  - Bronchoscopy biopsy forceps
  - Mucosal biopsy rarely carried out as the mucosa is very tough
  - Transbronchial biopsy not recommended as it is hazardous and of doubtful use in dogs and cats
- Lung biopsy
  - Fine needle aspirate
    - Well-defined mass lesions close to chest wall
    - Pleural effusions
    - Little value in diffuse lung disease
    - Can be carried out under ultrasound guidance
- Trucut biopsy of intrathoracic mass lesions

  - Submitted in formalin for histopathology
  - Usually best carried out by ultrasound guidance
  - Use large–gauge Trucut needles, e.g. 14G
- Open-chest biopsy
  - Major surgical procedure
  - Mainly carried out during exploratory thoracotomy
  - Immense diagnostic value, but technically difficult, hazardous and high level of morbidity (high-quality postoperative care required)
- Video-assisted thoracoscopic biopsy
  - Limited use in veterinary medicine
  - Specialist referral centres
  - Has potential, as it is less invasive and carries reduced morbidity
  - Benefits from detailed imaging information of suspected disease (e.g. computed tomography)

INVESTIGATION OF THE
CARDIORESPIRATORY CASE

SECTION 2
CARDIORESPIRATORY SYNDROMES

There are several clearly-recognised syndromes associated with diseases of the cardiopulmonary system, and in this section each of these clinical presentations are outlined. Additional detail regarding physical examination and diagnostic techniques are covered in Section 1 and in relevant sections throughout the book. To avoid repetition the reader is referred to these sections.

6 HEART FAILURE

Heart failure is a clinical syndrome – not a disease. Heart disease may be present without heart failure, but heart failure cannot be present without disease. Heart failure (HF) is the most common clinical presentation of dogs and cats with heart disease. It can be defined as a failure of the heart to circulate enough blood to meet the metabolic demands of the body at normal filling pressures. Congestive heart failure (CHF) infers that there is a damming back of blood behind the failing heart, into the pulmonary or systemic circulations.

MECHANISMS LEADING TO HEART FAILURE

The mechanisms that lead to HF can be described as being of four basic types.

PRESSURE OVERLOAD

- When the ventricle must generate increased pressure to overcome the resistance against which it ejects blood in order to maintain cardiac output
- Ventricle develops a compensatory concentric hypertrophy (myocardium becomes thicker without an increase in radius)
- Examples: aortic stenosis, pulmonic stenosis, systemic hypertension
- A pressure overload results in signs of forward failure and rarely congestive failure

VOLUME OVERLOAD

- Occurs when there is an increase in the volume of blood
- The myocardium adapts by dilating so that a greater volume of blood can be ejected with each contraction – compensatory eccentric hypertrophy
- Examples: mitral valve regurgitation, left-to-right cardiac shunts, excessive i/v fluids in cats

- A volume overload results in signs of congestive heart failure (as well as forward failure)

ABNORMALITIES IN CONTRACTILITY

- In dilated cardiomyopathy (DCM) the myocardium is unable to generate sufficient pressure to maintain cardiac output
- In hypertrophic cardiomyopathy (HCM) there is an excessive growth in muscle cells which results in a marked reduction in the chamber volume, significantly reducing diastolic filling and greatly reducing stroke volume
- Results in signs of congestive failure as well as forward failure

ABNORMALITIES OF RELAXATION (DIASTOLIC ABNORMALITIES)

- When there is a mechanical restriction to ventricular filling
- Examples: pericardial effusion causes cardiac tamponade, tachycardia-induced myocardial failure

CLINICAL MANIFESTATIONS OF HEART FAILURE

Forward and congestive (backward) heart failure are terms often used in describing heart failure. For the presentation and clinical signs of animals with heart failure see Chapter 1.

FORWARD FAILURE

- Forward failure refers to the inability of the heart to pump blood in a forward direction, i.e. out through the aorta, resulting in reduced peripheral perfusion
- Right-sided forward failure of the heart will result in a decreased return of blood to the left side, also resulting in forward failure
- Occasionally, reduced blood supply to the lungs (right-sided forward failure, e.g. pulmonic stenosis, tetralogy of Fallot) may be seen on thoracic radiographs as a hypovascular lung field

CONGESTIVE HEART FAILURE (CHF)

- Congestive failure refers to the damning back of blood behind the failing heart, hence it is sometimes referred to as backward failure. This has different effects depending upon whether it is behind the left or right sides of the heart.

Left-sided congestive failure

Left-sided CHF results in increased pulmonary venous pressures and ultimately pulmonary oedema.

Causes of left-sided congestive failure
- Mitral valve disease (myxomatous degeneration)
- Dilated cardiomyopathy in dogs
- Hypertrophic or restrictive cardiomyopathy in cats
- Congenital defects: mitral valve dysplasia, ventricular septal defect, patent ductus arteriosus

Note: In cats, left-sided congestive heart failure may result in pleural effusion.

Right-sided congestive failure

Right-sided CHF results in increased pressure in the vena cava, jugular distension, liver congestion, ascites and pleural effusion.

Causes of right-sided congestive failure
- Pericardial effusion and cardiac tamponade
- Tricuspid valve disease (myxomatous degeneration)
- Pulmonary hypertension (cor pulmonale)
- Heartworm disease (caval syndrome)
- Congenital defects: tricuspid valve dysplasia, tetralogy of Fallot, reverse shunting defects

Left- and right-sided (bilateral) congestive failure

There are a number of heart diseases that lead to both left and right sided congestive failure:
- Mitral and tricuspid valve disease (myxomatous degeneration)
- Dilated cardiomyopathy
- Hypertrophic or restrictive cardiomyopathy in cats

NEUROHORMONAL RESPONSE IN HEART FAILURE

Heart failure triggers complex, multiple, pathophysiological processes with activation of various neurohormonal systems such as:

- Sympathetic nervous system
- Renin–angiotensin system
- Aldosterone system
- Vasopressinergic system – antidiuretic hormone (ADH)
- Endothelin

- Atrial natriuretic peptide (ANP)
- Brain natriuretic peptide (BNP)
- Nitric oxide
- Cytokines

The goals of treatment are to alleviate the clinical signs of heart failure (improve quality of life) and to increase longevity by modifying these various deleterious neurohormonal compensatory mechanisms, in part with anti-neurohormonal drugs.

THERAPY

AIMS

The aims of therapy, which apply to most causes of congestive heart failure (except pericardial effusion), are as follows:

Control volume load (congestive signs)

- Diuretics – should be used at the minimum effective dose
  - Furosemide – the most potent and commonly used diuretic
  - Spironolactone – a weak diuretic but one with additional anti-aldosterone effects
  - Co-amilozide (hydrochlorothiazide + amiloride) – normally used in addition to furosemide when there is refractory ascites. This combination of diuretics acts at different sites within the nephron: the concept of *sequential nephron blockade.*
- ACE inhibitors
  - Have mild diuretic properties in addition to anti-neurohormonal effects
- Low-sodium diet
  - Excessive salt intake may exacerbate the fluid retention that occurs in heart failure and it is therefore generally agreed that high-salt diets and salty treats should be avoided

- Remove fluids
  - Drainage of pleural and/or ascitic fluid – usually performed only when fluid is causing dyspnoea, but removal also removes proteins and potentially reduces oncotic forces which could exacerbate oedema fluid
- Restriction of water intake
  - This is not advised and water should be provided ad lib

Reduce cardiac work

- Rest
  - Cage rest is important, especially in fulminant congestive failure cases
  - If oxygen administration causes stress, it should be avoided: consider hands-free methods, e.g. oxygen cage, anaesthetic chamber
  - Once congestive failure signs are controlled, exercise (within the limits of the animal's ability) is considered beneficial, but prevent excessive exercise
- Reduce arterial pressure (afterload)
  - Arterial vasodilators
    - Pimobendan – useful in acute fulminant cases; positive inotrope
    - Hydralazine – should be used judiciously and with careful monitoring
    - ACE inhibitor drugs – vasodilator benefits are mild and more long term

- Reduce the filling pressure (preload)
  - Venodilators
    - Diuretics – furosemide reduces pre-load, but is also reported to have venodilator properties when given i/v
    - Glyceryl trinitrate
    - Pimobendan
    - ACE inhibitors (mild)
- Weight reduction in obese animals
  - Obesity is a recognised cause of increased cardiac workload, especially during exercise

Improve cardiac efficiency

When myocardial failure is present.

- Enhance contractility with positive inotropic drugs:
  - Pimobendan
  - Digoxin
  - Dobutamine

- Improve diastolic function
  - Improve ventricular relaxation
    - Calcium channel blockers and β blockers may be useful in hypertrophic cardiomyopathy
  - Control arrhythmias such as:
    - Atrial fibrillation – digoxin would be the most commonly preferred drug
    - Frequent supraventricular premature complexes or ventricular premature complexes
- Improve myocardial or vascular remodelling
  - Counter the neurohormonal effects
    - ACE inhibitors
    - Angiotensin receptor antagonists
    - Beta blockers
    - Aldosterone antagonists, e.g. spironolactone

TREATMENT STRATEGIES

Treatment guidelines are also provided in each chapter discussing the disease. These guidelines provide a brief overview.

ACUTE FULMINANT CONGESTIVE FAILURE (PULMONARY OEDEMA)

Pulmonary oedema can occur in any dog or cat with rapidly progressing or uncontrolled congestive failure, but some common causes of acute failure are:

- Ruptured *chordae tendineae* secondary to mitral valve disease
- Acute onset dilated cardiomyopathy, particularly Dobermanns and Cocker Spaniels
- Cardiomyopathies in cats can present acutely, and may be associated with recent steroid administration or a salt load

Rest

- Strict rest and stress-free handling – cannot be over emphasised
- Gentle sedation results in:
  - Reduction in anxiety
  - Slower, deeper respiration
  - Dogs: morphine at 0.1–0.2 mg/kg i/m
  - Cats: butorphanol at 0.1 mg/kg i/m

Oxygen supplementation

- Without stressing the animal, using hands-free methods

Furosemide

- 4 mg/kg in dogs and 2 mg/kg in cats
- Administered i/v if it is not stressful to the animal, otherwise i/m
- Given every 1–2 hours until there is evidence of:
  - diuresis (urination)
  - improvement in respiration (reduction in pulmonary oedema)
  - at which time the frequency of administration is reduced to every six hours

> **Note:** Excessive dosing can potentially be counterproductive and may result in:
> - Dehydration
> - Reduced cardiac output
> - Circulatory collapse
> - Electrolyte depletion
> - Renal failure

Venodilators

Essentially redistribute blood volume away from the lungs to the large capacitance veins, thereby reducing pulmonary oedema

- *Sodium nitroprusside* – 1.0–5.0 µg/kg/min, preferably combined with dobutamine
  - Titrated upwards to effect, monitoring clinical response, systemic blood pressure (not less than 70 mmHg) and pulmonary capillary wedge pressure
  - Adverse effects include: hypotension, tachycardia, nausea and vomiting
- *Glyceryl trinitrate* – 0.5–5.0 cm in dogs tid, 0.5 cm in cats tid/qid
  - Simpler to use than sodium nitroprusside, although may be less effective
  - Applied to a hairless part of the body: inner ear or inside thigh (not rubbed in)

Caution: Need to use gloves when using, or handling dog.

Positive inotropes

- Beneficial in dogs with dilated cardiomyopathy, but also useful in dogs in acute failure due to mitral valve disease. Generally not used in cats in acute failure.
- *Dobutamine* – 5–10 µg/kg/min, usually combined with sodium nitroprusside
  - Titrated upwards to effect
  - See Table 6.1 for a simplified continuous rate infusion (CRI) calculation
- *Pimobendan* – 0.1–0.3 mg/kg bid po (on an empty stomach)
  - Simpler to use than dobutamine
  - Additionally provides arterial and venous vasodilation
  - Absorbed rapidly from gut
- *Digoxin* – not normally used as an emergency drug
  - It is a weak positive inotrope
  - Steady-state levels take 5–7 days to achieve, which is not appropriate in emergency cases
  - The intravenous preparation is difficult to use and has a narrow margin of safety

---

Summary of treatment strategies for the management of acute fulminant congestive heart failure in dogs

Option 1 – Intensive therapy
- Rest
- Gentle sedation
- Oxygen supplementation

TABLE 6.1 Calculation of constant rate infusion for dobutamine [replace 20 ml of 500 ml bag of fluids with 20 ml of dobutamine (12.5 mg/ml)]

Body Weight (kg)		10	20	30	40	50
Dose Rate (µg/kg/min)	Fluid Rate (ml/h)					
5		6	12	18	24	30
7.5		9	18	27	36	45
10		12	24	36	48	60

- Furosemide
- Sodium nitroprusside CRI
- Dobutamine CRI

Option 2 – Less intensive
More likely to be an option in general practice
- Rest
- Gentle sedation
- Oxygen supplementation
- Furosemide i/v or i/m
- Glyceryl trinitrate percutaneous
- Pimobendan po

Summary of treatment of acute pulmonary oedema in cats due to hypertrophic or restrictive cardiomyopathy

- Rest – cage rest is particularly beneficial in cats
- Gentle sedation
- Oxygen supplementation
- Furosemide – 2 mg/kg every two hours, until an improvement in signs
- Glyceryl trinitrate $1/4''$ tid

Note: Pleural effusion, if present, will require drainage.

CHRONIC CONGESTIVE FAILURE (OUT-PATIENT TREATMENT) IN DOGS

The majority of heart failure patients will fall into this category.
- The general rule is that treatment should not be initiated until there are clinical signs
- Exercise is considered important, but should be well within the capabilities of the patient

ACE inhibitors

Indicated in all dogs with heart failure due to mitral valve disease or dilated cardiomyopathy because of the importance of inhibiting the adverse neuroendocrine

responses that are induced by CHF. Being increasingly used in cats.
- There are a large number of ACE inhibitors available, none has a particular advantage or benefit compared to others
- Start at standard manufacturer recommended dose
- Dose can be doubled to bid in long standing or advanced cases

Diuretics

- Dose should be adjusted and optimised in each case

Furosemide
- Dose range is 1–4 mg/kg bid in dogs, 1–2 mg/kg sid/bid in cats
- Initial dose is proportional to severity of disease
- Oral furosemide solution is often a more convenient medication for cats and more accurately titrated when the dose is small
- Following a response, the dose should be reduced to the minimum effective dose
- In many cats, without concurrent pleural effusion, the furosemide can often be weaned off, the animals being maintained on an ACE inhibitor

Note: Diuretic over dosage can lead to: subclinical dehydration, inappetance, lethargy, pre-renal azotaemia, depletion of electrolytes, polydipsia/polyuria.

Atrial fibrillation (AF) control

- Important when the ventricular response rate exceeds 150/min
- May not be necessary in giant-breed dog with lone AF

Digoxin (Also see p. 77)
- The most commonly used drug
- Primarily used in dogs; indications for use in the cat are rare and not discussed

- Dose – 0.22 mg/m^2 every 12 hours – Table 6.2 provides a simple guideline for starting dose
- Steady state levels are achieved in 5–7 days
- Serum digoxin levels should be measured (approximately six hours post pill, day 5–7) to confirm the dose is correct, as it varies between individual patients
- Therapeutic serum levels are 0.8–2.5 ng/ ml; 1–2 ng/mg is a reasonable target
- Therapeutic aim is to reduce the heart rate to less than 150–160/min, however judging the heart rate in-clinic may result in falsely high heart rates, so clinical judgement needs to be made or Holter monitoring considered
- Bioaccumulation of digoxin may occur with azotaemia, low serum albumin, cachexia
- Signs of over dosage are: depression, anorexia, vomiting/diarrhoea, arrhythmias, in which case the drug should be stopped and re-introduced at a lower dose when signs have completely resolved.

Causes of a persistent high heart rate in dogs with AF receiving digoxin
- Elevation of the heart rate in-clinic due to nervousness at the time of examination – may require 24-hour Holter to determine average heart rate at home
- Inadequate control of the congestive failure signs – sympathetic drive is still high
- Dehydration/hypotension due to over-diuresis/vasodilation

- Inadequate serum therapeutic levels of digoxin
- Concurrent medical disease, e.g. renal failure
- Advanced myocardial failure and end-stage heart disease
- Heart rate poorly responsive to digoxin – needs additional antiarrhythmic drugs

Positive inotropic drugs

Digoxin is a weak positive inotrope that has been superseded by pimobendan.

> **Note:** Digoxin and pimobendan can be used simultaneously in a dog.

Indications
- Dogs with dilated cardiomyopathy
- Dogs with mitral valve disease in which there is myocardial failure
- May be of benefit in cats with cardiomyopathy where there is reduced wall motion

Pimobendan
- 0.1–0.3 mg/kg bid, on an empty stomach
- Also has arterial vasodilator properties
- Positive lusitropic properties (improves relaxation)
- Additional effects are: improvement in the animal's demeanour, alertness and activity and sometimes an improvement in appetite
- Inhibits platelet aggregation

Note: Calcium channel antagonists may reduce the efficacy of pimobendan.

TABLE 6.2 Digoxin starting dose in dogs

Body Weight (kg)	Tablet Strength (µg)	Tablet Dose (bid)
1–5	62.5 (PG)	$^1/_2$
6–13	62.5 (PG)	1
14–23	125	1
24–36	125	$1^1/_2$
>37	250	1

Summary of treatment strategy for treatment of chronic congestive heart failure (out-patient treatment) in dogs

- Exercise – within animal's capability
- ACE inhibitor (ACE I)
- Furosemide – to minimum effective dose
- Digoxin – primarily in cases with atrial fibrillation
- Pimobendan – in dogs with myocardial failure.

CHRONIC CONGESTIVE HEART FAILURE (OUT-PATIENT TREATMENT) IN CATS

- Exercise – within animal's capability
- ACE inhibitor
- Furosemide – to minimum effective dose
- Beta blockers or calcium channel blockers may be of additional benefit in cats with hypertrophic obstructive cardiomyopathy (see Chapter 11, p. 108)
- Pimobendan – might be of benefit in cats with cardiomyopathy where there is reduced wall motion (a similar dose to dogs can be used, but it is not licensed for use in cats)

REFRACTORY CHRONIC HEART FAILURE IN DOGS (OFTEN WITH ASCITES)

Refractory heart failure occurs primarily in dogs with dilated cardiomyopathy, but is seen eventually in dogs with mitral and tricuspid valve disease.

- Ascites (+/– pleural effusion) becomes refractory to the above treatment, including top doses of furosemide (4 mg/kg bid)

- In these cases the dose of ACE inhibitors should be doubled to bid and the dose of pimobendan maximised
- If ascites remains refractory then additional diuresis is required
  - Spironolactone at 1–2 mg/kg bid
    - Beneficial anti-aldosterone properties, reduction in myocardial fibrosis
    - A weak but potassium-sparing diuretic
  - Co-amilozide (hydrochlorothiazide + amiloride) at 1–3 mg/kg bid (combined dose rate)
    - A more potent and useful diuretic
    - Amiloride is a potassium-sparing diuretic

> **Note:** There is some interest in the use of spironolactone at sub-diuretic doses ($^1/_4$ normal dose), as part of the treatment regime, to minimise/reduce myocardial fibrosis.

REFRACTORY CHRONIC HEART FAILURE IN CATS (WITH PLEURAL EFFUSION)

Persistent pleural effusion is not an uncommon problem in cats with heart disease and the prognosis for these cases is quite poor.

- Initial management involves thoracocentesis, at the minimum draining sufficient fluid to relieve any dyspnoea.
- Most cats will then require ongoing diuretics, e.g. furosemide 1–2 mg/kg sid or bid, in addition to an ACE inhibitor.
- Combination diuretics can be tried, but diuretic side effects become more problematic (more so in cats than dogs), thus intermittent thoracocentesis may also be required.

7 ARRHYTHMIAS

- Arrhythmias are a frequent finding in cardiac disease but are also often secondary to systemic diseases
- Cats have a lower incidence of arrhythmias than dogs

- A basic understanding of electrophysiology and its mechanisms is necessary to understand management and treatment
- See also Chapter 3, Electrocardiography

ABNORMALITIES IN RATE AND CONDUCTION

SINUS BRADYCARDIA

Causes
- May be a normal variation in athletically fit animals
- Hypothyroidism
- Hyperkalaemia
- Hypothermia
- Elevated intracranial pressure
- Systemic disease (e.g. renal failure)
- Drugs (tranquillisers or antiarrhythmic drugs)

Treatment
- Should be aimed at the primary cause
- Vagolytic or beta-agonist drugs can be used to increase the heart rate if symptomatic

SINUS TACHYCARDIA

Sinus tachycardia is a non-specific rhythm disturbance.

Causes
- Heart failure (due to a compensatory sympathetic drive)
- Physiological response (e.g. stress, excitement, fear)

- Systemic disease (e.g. pyrexia, pain, anaemia, dehydration)

Treatment
Treatment should be aimed at the primary cause, usually negating the need to use antiarrhythmic drugs

> **Note:** In animals in congestive heart failure, sinus tachycardia is often a necessary compensatory response in an attempt to maintain cardiac output, So antiarrhythmic drugs are generally not used to slow the heart rate. Treatment is instead directed towards the congestive failure (see Chapter 6), following which the heart rate then slows as sympathetic drive reduces.

SINUS ARREST/BLOCK

Sinus arrest/block can be a normal finding in some brachycephalic dogs (i.e. exaggerated respiratory sinus arrhythmia).

Differentials
- Sick sinus syndrome (sinus node dysfunction)

- Irritation of the vagus nerve
  - Neoplasia in the cervical area (e.g. thyroid carcinoma)
  - Neoplasia in the thorax (e.g. aortic body tumour)
- Vagal stimulation associated with severe respiratory disease or vomiting
- Atrial disease (e.g. dilation, fibrosis, cardiomyopathy, neoplasia, drug toxicity, electrolyte imbalance, hypothyroidism)

Treatment

Treatment is usually only required in symptomatic cases. Pacemaker implantation is often the treatment of choice.

SICK SINUS SYNDROME (SINUS NODE DYSFUNCTION)

- In the bradycardia-tachycardia syndrome either the bradycardia or the tachycardia may cause syncope
- Most commonly seen in West Highland White Terriers (with or without idiopathic pulmonary fibrosis)
- Also reported in older, female miniature Schnauzers
- Not recorded in cats
- Profound sinus bradycardia and sinus arrest are usually the main causes of clinical signs such as:
  - Lethargy
  - Exercise intolerance
  - Weakness
  - Collapse/syncope
- If atropine or exercise fail to increase the heart rate significantly (see Box below), it indicates that excessive vagal tone is not the cause of the bradycardia
- Symptomatic cases may require pacemaker implantation, and possibly antiarrhythmic drugs

> **Atropine response test**
> Inject 40 µg/kg s/c (dog and cat) and re-assess heart-rate response (ECG) in 30–40 minutes.

ATRIAL STANDSTILL

- Rule out the presence of small P waves by use of chest leads
  - Confirm absence of atrial activity on echocardiography
    - Mitral/tricuspid valve motion on M-mode
    - Mitral/tricuspid inflow velocities on Doppler studies
- Atropine does not increase the heart rate
- The prognosis is usually poor

Associated conditions

- Facioscapulohumeral muscular dystrophy in English Springer Spaniels and Old English Sheepdogs
- Hyperkalaemia
- Atrial cardiomyopathy in dogs

Clinical signs

- Weakness
- Lethargy
- Syncope
- Congestive heart failure

Treatment

Treatment is directed towards congestive heart failure if present and some patients may benefit from pacemaker implantation.

AV BLOCK

Clinical signs associated with advanced second degree or complete AV block

- Weakness
- Exercise intolerance

- Lethargy
- Syncope
- Sudden death

Causes

- Idiopathic (most common cause) – fibrosis of the AV node
- Cardiomyopathy
- Cardiac neoplasia
- Endocarditis
- Digitalis toxicity
- Hyperkalemia

Treatment

Treatment may be attempted with:
- Parasympatholytic drugs
  - Atropine – Dog/cat: 40 µg/kg s/c or i/v
  - Propantheline –
    Dog: 0.5–2 mg/kg q8–12h po;
    Cat: 7.5 mg q8–12h po
- Sympathomimetic drugs
  - Clenbuterol –
    Dog: 1–5 µg/kg q8–12h;
    Cat 1 µg/kg q12–24h
  - Terbutaline – 1.25–5 mg/dog q8h; 1.25 mg/cat q8h
- Millophyline may be of some help in cats, or theophylline in dogs
- Pacemaker implantation is often necessary

ABNORMALITIES DUE TO ECTOPIA

VENTRICULAR ARRHYTHMIAS

- Ventricular premature complexes (VPCs) may occur due to
  - Primary heart disease
    - Cardiomyopathies (e.g. dilated, hypertrophic, restrictive, arrhythmogenic)
    - Congestive heart failure (+/– hypokalaemia, hypomagnesaemia)
    - Myocarditis
    - Cardiac neoplasia
    - Endocarditis
    - Congenital ventricular arrhythmias in German Shepherd pups
    - Magnesium deficiency syndrome of growth in giant-breed, rapidly-growing pups
  - Secondary to a systemic disorder
    - gastric dilation/volvulus
    - pancreatitis
    - splenic masses
    - electrolyte imbalance
    - cranial trauma (brain-heart syndrome)
    - low blood oxygen saturation
- Treatment of the primary underlying cause (e.g. congestive heart failure) will often produce a significant reduction in VPCs, thus in many cases institution of antiarrhythmic drug treatment should be postponed to see if this occurs
- A ventricular arrhythmia is considered significant when it causes haemodynamic compromise and thus signs such as:
  - Pallor
  - Exercise intolerance
  - Systemic hypotension
  - Weakness/recumbency
  - Syncope
- Indications for treatment are listed below
- True frequency of serious arrhythmias may only be detected by 24-hour Holter monitoring
  - <200 VPCs per 24 hours is considered a low frequency
  - >1000 VPCs per 24 hours is considered a high frequency
- In Dobermanns, a sustained ventricular tachycardia (VT), >30 seconds, is considered a predictor of sudden death

CARDIORESPIRATORY SYNDROMES

Indications for antiarrhythmic drug treatment of ventricular arrhythmias

- Frequent multimorphic VPCs
- VPCs with a very short coupling interval, i.e. R-on-T
- Rapid sustained VT (>150/min)
- Frequent VPCs or VT in Boxers and Dobermanns (with cardiomyopathy)
- VT with inherited ventricular arrhythmias of German Shepherd Dogs (<18 months of age)

Treatment

Aims of antiarrhythmic drug treatment are to reduce risk of sudden death and/or improve clinical signs. However some studies have shown that antiarrhythmic drugs have the potential to cause sudden death, thus their use needs strong justification.

- In most circumstances institution of antiarrhythmics orally is satisfactory
- If VPCs are life threatening, i/v *lidocaine* is the drug of choice (see below)
- Response to treatment can be assessed from Holter monitoring pre and post treatment. A significant response to an antiarrhythmic drug is considered to be a reduction in VPCs by 75% when the VPCs are frequent
- Following cardioversion of a ventricular arrhythmia with lidocaine, the options are:
  ○ Wait and see if the arrhythmia does return (in which case repeat cardioversion is required)
  ○ Administer i/v lidocaine as a constant rate infusion (Table 7.1)
  ○ Usual starting dose is 50 μg/kg/min

Note: Steady state levels take 3–6 hours to reach, so small boluses of lidocaine may be required in the interim
  ○ Medicate with an oral antiarrhythmic such as mexiletine (which seems a pragmatic approach)

Lidocaine (lignocaine)

- Drug of choice for the cardioversion of acute, life-threatening, ventricular tachycardia
- Its effects are nullified in the presence of hypokalaemia
- Following i/v administration the half-life is approximately 60–90 minutes and antiarrhythmic effects wane after ten minutes
- If i/v lidocaine proves ineffective then alternative i/v options are *esmolol* and *procainamide*

Dosage

- Dog: Bolus doses at 2–3 mg/kg slowly i/v every few minutes, to a maximum of 9 mg/kg
- Cat: Slow i/v at 0.25–0.75 mg/kg; may give a repeat i/v injection after 20 minutes

Note: Cats are very sensitive and prone to toxic side effects (seizures and respiratory arrest).

Table 7.1 Calculation of constant rate infusion for lidocaine (replace 25 ml of 500 ml bag of fluids with 25 ml of 2% lidocaine without adrenaline [21 mg/ml])

Body Weight (kg)		10	20	30	40	50
Dose Rate (μg/kg/min)	Fluid Rate (ml/h)					
25		15	30	45	60	75
50		30	60	90	120	150
70		45	90	135	180	225

Toxicity

- Signs of toxicity are *neurological* (twitching, nystagmus, seizures), these are usually self-limiting, and *gastrointestinal* (nausea, vomiting, salivation)
- Airway obstruction and/or respiratory arrest in cats following seizures
- Control seizures with i/v diazepam – 0.1 mg/kg i/v; repeat every few minutes to effect, to a maximum of 0.5 mg/kg; elevate head

Other antiarrhythmic drugs

- Mexiletine
  - One of the most common antiarrhythmics used in dogs
  - Recommended for VT in the inherited ventricular arrhythmia of GSDs
  - Similar properties to lidocaine
  - If lidocaine cardioverts an arrhythmia successfully, mexiletine is often effective when used to maintain control
  - Dose in dog: 5–8 mg/kg q8h po
  - If mexiletine provides insufficient control, add atenolol (useful in treatment of Boxers with VT)
- Propranolol – Dog: 0.2–2.0 mg/kg q8h; Cat: 2.5 mg q8–12h
- Atenolol – Dog: 0.25–2.0 mg/kg q12h po (start at lowest dose); Cat: 1–2 mg/kg q12–24h
- Sotalol – Dog: 0.5–2.0 mg/kg q12h (often used in Boxers with VT)
- Amiodarone (dogs)
  - Reported to have significant side effects, so tends to be used as a last resort
  - Need to monitor liver and thyroid function regularly
  - Loading dose: 10–15 mg/kg q12h po for 5–10 days
  - Maintenance dose: 5–10 mg/kg q24hr (to minimum effective dose)
- Magnesium deficiency syndrome of growth
  - Magnesium amino chelate (200 mg tablets) at 10 mg/kg daily with food

- Beta blockers are the main drugs used to control ventricular arrhythmias in cats

> **Note:** Most antiarrhythmic drugs have a negative inotropic effect and should be used with caution in dogs with myocardial failure.

Ventricular arrhythmias associated with gastric dilation/volvulus (GDV)

Approximately 40–50% of dogs with gastric dilation volvulus (GDV) develop ventricular arrhythmias 12–72 hours after the onset of GDV.

Causes

- Myocardial ischaemia (decreased coronary perfusion)
- Reperfusion injury
- Hypokalaemia (can also make the arrhythmias resistant to antiarrhythmic drugs)
- Acidosis
- Hypoxia
- Myocardial depressant factors

Treatment

Treatment is directed towards:
- Shock
- Maintenance of normal hydration status
- Correction of acid–base and electrolyte imbalances
- Monitoring Na^+ and K^+ regularly in such cases is very useful as hypokalaemia is a common problem (although measurement of serum K^+ may not reflect total body K^+)

SUPRAVENTRICULAR ARRHYTHMIAS

Supraventricular premature complexes (SVPCs) and *supraventricular tachycardia*

(SVT) commonly occur as a result of atrial wall stretching.

Causes
- Congenital or acquired AV valve disease
- Cardiomyopathy
- Congenital cardiac shunts
- Right atrial haemangiosarcoma
- Digoxin toxicity (SVT is usually <160/min in dogs)
- Hyperthyroidism in cats
- Abnormal accessory pathways can also lead to primary rhythm disturbances
- Re-entrant SVT – in dogs most are bypass tract macro-re-entrant, rather than AV nodal (Wolff-Parkinson-White syndrome)

Clinical signs
- Clinical signs can be caused by very frequent SVPCs or sustained SVT, and include:
  - Weakness
  - Ataxia (presyncope)
  - Collapse
  - Tachypnoea
- Signs are more severe when there is underlying organic heart disease
- When an SVT is maintained at high rate (>250/min) for days or weeks it can result in tachycardia-induced myocardial failure (see Chapter 12) and congestive heart failure

Treatment
- The aims of treatment:
  - SVT – cardiovert to a normal sinus rhythm and maintain control
  - SVPCs – reduce frequency
- Treatment should be directed to any underlying disease first, particularly when there is organic heart disease
- Vagal manoeuvres such as carotid sinus massage – Up and down moving pressure applied behind the angle of the jaw for ten seconds
  - May terminate an SVT

- May slow an SVT and help identify the type of arrhythmia
- May be ineffectual when animals have a high sympathetic tone, such as when they are nervous or in heart failure
- May work better after administration of beta-blockers or calcium channel antagonists
- In a dog with sustained SVT or collapse, i/v cardioversion is necessary

Antiarrhythmic drugs
Intravenous antiarrhythmic drugs
- Verapamil – calcium channel antagonist
  - Dose in dog: 0.05 mg/kg i/v every five minutes to effect (maximum 0.15 mg/kg in 10–15 min)
- Esmolol – short-acting beta-blocker with a half-life of nine minutes
  - Dose in dog: 0.05–0.10 mg/kg slow i/v q5 min to a maximum of 0.5 mg/kg
- Lidocaine – may have effects on some macro-re-entrant SVTs and is worth trying if other drugs fail
  - 2–3 mg/kg, repeated every few minutes to response, up to a maximum of 9 mg/kg
- Procainamide – 2 mg/kg i/v, repeated to response, up to a maximum of 15 mg/kg in 20 minutes

Oral antiarrhythmic drugs
- Calcium antagonists
  - Diltiazem – Dog: 1–3 mg/kg q8h (start at lowest dose); Cat: 1.6–3.3 mg/kg q8h po; slow release (Dilacor XR) 30 mg/cat q24h
  - Verapamil – Dog: 0.05 mg/kg i/v q5min to effect (maximum 0.15 mg/kg in 10–15 min); Cat: 0.025 mg/kg i/v
- beta-blockers
  - Atenolol – Dog: 0.25–2 mg/kg q12h po
  - Propranolol – Dog: 0.2–2 mg/kg q8hr po (start at lowest dose)

Note: When stopping beta-blockers, patients should be weaned off slowly.

- Digoxin
  - Onset of action is too slow
  - Dose: see Atrial fibrillation below
- Sotalol
  - Dose in dog: 0.5–2 mg/kg q12h
- Amiodarone (dog)
  - Reported to have significant side effects, so tends to be used as a last resort
  - Need to monitor liver and thyroid function regularly
  - Loading dose: 10–15 mg/kg q12h po for 5–10 days
  - Maintenance dose: 5–10 mg/kg q24h (use minimum effective dose)

FIBRILLATION AND FLUTTER

Ventricular fibrillation (VF)

- Causes are numerous, but similar to those of VPCs and VT
- Treatment is initiation of cardiopulmonary resuscitation with electrical defibrillation (see Chapter 20), however the success of this will depend on the extent of existing pathology

Atrial fibrillation and flutter

- Loss of the atrial contraction contribution to cardiac output is approximately 20%. This is compensated for by an increase in stroke volume and rate.
- Usually occurs as a result of underlying organic pathology, i.e. dilation of one or both atria.
- May occur without existing atrial pathology in large and giant breed dogs – referred to as *lone AF* (although most do progress to dilated cardiomyopathy).
- It is rare in the cat, but may be seen when there is severe left atrial dilation with hypertrophic or restrictive cardiomyopathy.
- If the heart rate with AF is not fast (<120–130/min), as with lone AF in giant-breed dogs, then the use of drugs

to further control the rate is debatable. However, β-blockers may be useful to minimise tachycardia during periods of high sympathetic tone, such as exercise or stress, and may have long-term benefits (upregulation of beta receptors) in occult DCM.

- Cardioversion of atrial fibrillation to sinus rhythm is generally not attempted because there is usually cardiac pathology.
- The drug of choice for rate control of AF is usually digoxin because of its mild positive inotropic properties.
- If there is good myocardial function, then calcium antagonists or β-blockers are alternative options – however these should be used with caution in dogs with myocardial failure.

Use of digoxin for rate control of AF

- Primarily used in dogs; indications for use in cat are rare
- Dose in dog: 0.22 mg/m^2 every 12 hours; Table 6.2, p. 69, provides a simple guideline for a starting dose

Note: Dobermann dose is 125 μg bid.

- Dose in cat: <4 kg – 0.0625 mg tablet 1/2 q48 hours; >4 kg – 0.0625 mg tablet 1/2 q24 hours
- Steady-state levels are achieved in 5–7 days
- Serum digoxin levels should be measured (approximately six hours post pill) to confirm the dose is correct, as it varies between individual patients
- Therapeutic dose range is 0.8–2.5 ng/ml, 1–2 ng/ml is a good target
- Therapeutic aim is to reduce the heart rate (at rest and non-stressed) to less than 150–160/min in dogs and <240/min in cats. Assessment of the heart rate in-clinic may result in falsely high heart rates, so clinical judgement needs to be made or Holter monitoring considered.
- Causes of a persistently high heart rate are listed below

- Bioaccumulation may occur with: azotaemia, low serum albumin, cachexia
- Signs of over-dosage are: depression, anorexia, vomiting/diarrhoea, arrhythmias, in which case the drug should be stopped and re-introduced at a lower dose when signs have completely resolved

Causes of a persistently high heart rate in dogs receiving digoxin for atrial fibrillation

- Elevation of the heart rate in-clinic due to nervousness at the time of examination
  - may require 24-hour Holter to determine average heart rate at home
- Inadequate control of the congestive failure signs – sympathetic drive is still high
- Dehydration/hypotension due to over-diuresis/vasodilation
- Inadequate serum levels of digoxin
- Concurrent medical disease, e.g. renal failure
- Advanced myocardial failure and end-stage heart disease
- Heart rate poorly responsive to digoxin – needs additional antiarrhythmic drugs

PACEMAKERS

INDICATIONS

Symptomatic bradyarrhythmias

- Complete AV block
- 2nd degree Mobitz type II, persistent or intermittent
- 2nd degree Mobitz type I, with symptoms
- Profound sinus bradycardia
- Sinus arrest
- 'Tachy-brady' sick sinus syndrome, when anti-tachyarrhythmia drugs produce symptoms
- AF or flutter with a slow ventricular response and symptoms (rare in dogs and cats)
- Persistent atrial standstill (questionable)

CONTRAINDICATIONS

- Active infection
- Dilated cardiomyopathy
- Cardiac neoplasia

Note: Bradyarrhythmia may be an early sign of cardiomyopathy and the long-term prognosis poor due to the underlying heart disease.

Complications

Complications are significantly reduced with cardiologists experienced in implantation (>20 implants)

Major complications
- Lead dislodgement
- Pacemaker failure, e.g. premature battery death
- Anaesthestic-related death – reduced by placement of a temporary pacing lead prior to induction of anaesthesia
- Infection of pulse generator/pouch
- Lead fracture
- Venous thrombosis and chylothorax in cats

Minor complications
- Seroma formation
- Muscle twitch
- Induced arrhythmias
- Pacemaker movement

Equipment

- Pacemaker
  ○ Contains electronic circuitry with lithium battery power source
  ○ Lasts 5–10 years
  ○ Unit is hermetically sealed in titanium housing
- Leads
  ○ *Unipolar*: the cathode (negative) is at

the distal tip and the anode (positive) is the pacemaker

○ *Bipolar*: the anode is 1 cm proximal to the cathode, in the form of a ring electrode; less sensitive to myopotential inhibition, and less likely to cause muscle twitch

○ *Tined* (passive) and *screw-in* (active) leads are available; there appear to be few advantages of one over the other

- Pacemaker system programmer/analyser – different for every manufacturer; the assistance of a local hospital ECG technician is essential
- Lead position guided by fluoroscopic image intensification
- External temporary pacemaker, used to assess minimum amount of current required to stimulate the ventricle, indicating good electrode to endocardial contact
- Post-surgical protective bandages to prevent dog scratching out sutures and introducing potentially lethal infection

TYPES OF PERMANENT PACEMAKER

The more commonly used pacemakers are:
- VVI – paces and senses in ventricle; inhibited by intrinsic ventricular beats (demand pacemaker).
- VVIR – additionally rate responsive (increase in rate) on detection of movement
  ○ VVI and VVIR are the common modes used in animals, as they require only one lead
- VDR – paces and senses the ventricle, but additionally there are sensors at atrial level; can track P waves (in AV block) and pace ventricles following each P wave, providing atrioventricular synchrony and sinus node rate control; available human leads are only suitable for very large-breed dogs

- DDD – has two leads and paces and senses both atrium and ventricle; atrial lead placement is difficult in dogs.

TECHNIQUES OF IMPLANTATION

- The transvenous (jugular) route is currently the preferred option. This involves the exposure of an external jugular vein, insertion of the pacing lead with fluoroscopic guidance, and placing the pulse generator subcutaneously in the dorsal neck. The jugular vein is normally occluded.
- Epicardial lead placement requires direct exposure of the left ventricular apex, and thus surgical intervention (e.g. thoracotomy or laparotomy), but does not require fluoroscopy.

PACEMAKER FOLLOW-UP

Owners should bring dogs for regular follow-up examinations and programming checks for potential problems.
- 3–4 months following implantation, programming check and reset current levels to minimise battery use
- Annual programming checks to ensure function and detect evidence of declining battery life

HAZARDS

- Pacemakers occasionally sense extrinsic electromagnetic interference (EMI), but with modern units this is minimised by pacemaker designs and shielding; surgical cautery and MRI are problems
- Disposal of a carcass: before this can be done, the pulse generator must be removed as cremation of the lithium battery results in explosion!

8 EPISODIC WEAKNESS AND COLLAPSE

- Brief episodes of weakness or collapse are seen fairly frequently in dogs (less so in cats) and present a diagnostic challenge particularly as they are often normal at the time of presentation. This chapter is primarily concerned with this type of case.
- It has been shown that a diagnosis can be made in approximately 50% of such cases. Of the remaining 50%, in which no diagnosis is made, approximately half resolve spontaneously and death or further deterioration are rare outcomes.
- The causes of collapse can be broadly categorised into: *syncope*, *weakness* and *seizures*.

SYNCOPE

- Syncope (fainting) is a sudden, transient loss of consciousness that occurs when cerebral blood flow falls. The reduced blood flow results in a deprivation of energy substrates (oxygen or glucose) which impairs cerebral metabolism.
- Often due to cardiovascular disease.
- It should be noted that an acute reduction in cardiac output causes mucous membrane pallor; in contrast cyanosis is more commonly associated with respiratory disease.

CAUSES OF SYNCOPE

- Vasovagal syncope (also known as *neurally mediated syncope*, *vasodepressor syncope* and *faint*)
  - Transient bradycardia and/or systemic hypotension
  - Triggered by a surge of catecholamines, such as with excitement or sudden exercise – a common cause of 'fainting' in Boxers (see below)
  - Tussive syncope – collapse follows a paroxysm of coughing
  - Micturition syncope – collapse follows straining to urinate
- Reduced cardiac output
  - Profound bradyarrhythmias, e.g. sinus arrest
  - Profound tachyarrhythmias, e.g. ventricular tachycardia
  - Acute forward failure on exertion
  - Inadequate cardiac output (forward failure) on exertion: dilated cardiomyopathy, hypertrophic obstructive cardiomyopathy, pericardial effusion, aortic stenosis, pulmonic stenosis
- Hypoxia
  - Hypoxia can occur with hypoventilation (upper airway obstruction), diffusion abnormalities and ventilation/perfusion mismatch as occurs with severe lung parenchymal disease or *cor pulmonale*
  - Cyanosis is often found with severe airway obstructive disorders such as laryngeal paralysis, tracheal collapse and brachycephalic upper airway syndrome
  - While right-to-left cardiac shunts are rare, they tend to produce cyanosis with polycythaemia

- ○ Anaemia or acute haemorrhage may lead to collapse, often easily recognised, but in some case an abdominal bleed can be quite subtle, e.g. haemorrhage due to a splenic haemangiosarcoma
- Hypoglycaemia
  - ○ Insulinoma
  - ○ Insulin overdose in a diabetic animal
  - ○ Working dog hypoglycaemia
  - ○ Other causes are much less common and include liver disease and sepsis

COLLAPSE IN BOXERS – SOME DIFFERENTIAL DIAGNOSES

- Vasovagal collapse
  - ○ Tends to occur in clusters in younger dogs following excitement/exertion

- Ventricular tachycardia
  - ○ Dilated cardiomyopathy
  - ○ Arrhythmogenic right ventricular cardiomyopathy
- Subaortic stenosis (severe)
  - ○ May cause output failure on exertion

PRE-SYNCOPE

Transient partial reduction in blood flow to the brain may result in an episode of weakness or ataxia rather than an absolute syncopal episode. For example:
- Rapid supraventricular tachycardia (SVT)
- Dilated cardiomyopathy
- Pericardial effusion

WEAKNESS

- *Weakness* is defined as a loss of muscular strength resulting in an animal becoming completely or partially recumbent or ataxic. Generalised muscle weakness is referred to as *asthenia*. Weakness can be continuous or episodic.
- Many conditions produce a continuing weakness due to advanced disease and the diagnosis is often more apparent (e.g. kidney or liver disease, haemorrhage).
- Heart failure also produces weakness (forward failure). On exertion or exercise the animal becomes weak and may become recumbent (appear to collapse).

CAUSES OF WEAKNESS

Neurological or neuromuscular disease
- Disorders of neuromuscular transmission
  - ○ Myasthenia gravis
- Myopathies

- ○ Polymyopathy or polymyositis
- ○ Labrador and Golden Retriever myopathy
- ○ Hypokalaemic polymyopathy in cats
- Exercise induced collapse (EIC) – see below
- Peripheral neuropathies
  - ○ Vestibular syndrome (sometimes erroneously referred to as a 'stroke')

Exercise induced collapse (EIC)
- Documented in Labrador Retrievers, but a similar condition occurs in Border Collies in the UK
- Affects excitable athletically fit young dogs
- Appears to be more prevalent in the warmer months of the year
- Whilst dogs can tolerate routine exercise, they struggle with episodes of strenuous/extreme exertion and become weak, recumbent and appear exhausted with excessive panting

- There may be ataxia and reduced proprioceptive deficits primarily of the hind legs
- Rectal temperature during a collapse is often >41°C and affected animals seek a cool resting place, although normal dogs also have a high temperature following marked exertion
- Recovery may take 5–20 minutes, during which time affected dogs remain mentally bright and alert
- No known treatment and limiting exercise is recommended

Non-cardiorespiratory medical conditions

A variety of medical conditions (e.g. endocrinopathies and metabolic diseases) can result in weakness and occasionally collapse.

- Hyperkalaemia – often results in bradyarrhythmias
  - Addison's disease
  - Diabetic ketoacidosis
  - Acute/oliguric renal failure
  - Obstructive urinary disorders
- Hypokalaemia
  - Polymyopathy in cats
- Hypocalcaemia
  - Post-parturient eclampsia
  - Hypoparathyroidism
- Hypothyroidism – may lead to bradyarrhythmias
- Hyperadrenocorticism
- Phaeochromocytoma
- Hyperthermia ('heat stroke')
- Polycythaemia
- Severe acid – base imbalance

SEIZURES

- Seizure (epilepsy, fit, convulsion) refers to an involuntary, paroxysmal and uncontrolled muscular activity due to a disturbance in the brain's activity.
- Seizures can be divided into generalised tonic ≠ clonic (grand mal) or partial seizures (petit mal). The latter can present as a transient loss of consciousness.
- The classical grand mal seizure is relatively easy to recognise – tonic/clonic contractions, defecation, a pre-ictal phase and post-ictal dementia or abnormal behaviour are often noted with generalised seizures.
  - Central nervous system (CNS) disorders
    - Hepatic encephalopathy
    - Narcolepsy or cataplexy
    - Scottie cramp
    - Episodic falling over in Cavalier King Charles Spaniels
- Partial seizures are relatively rare, but can mimic syncope.

> **Note:** It is possible for a syncopal animal to develop opisthotonus or seizure-like activity if cerebral hypoxia persists for some time (an *hypoxic seizure*). Detailed history taking should allow differentiation. Animals with a syncopal event are fairly motionless and flaccid at the *start* of the event in contrast to those with a seizure.

INVESTIGATION OF WEAKNESS OR COLLAPSE

HISTORY

The history should establish whether the animal has had a seizure or a syncopal episode. Since such episodes are rarely witnessed by the veterinary surgeon there is great reliance on the accuracy of the owner's report.

Pre-ictal phase

With seizures there is usually a change in character or behaviour immediately before the episode, but this rarely occurs in other causes of collapse.

Time of episode
- With cardiac and neuromuscular disorders syncope/weakness is associated with excitement, exercise, stress or sudden arousal from sleep.
- Hypoglycaemia or hepatic encephalopathy may have a reasonably constant relation to feeding time, i.e. just before or shortly after feeding.
- Seizures usually occur at rest or when sleeping and less frequently during activity or in an unfamiliar environment.

During the episode
Type of activity
- With seizures there is tonic/clonic movement of the limbs and jaw, tremor, salivation, tachypnoea and tachycardia, and involuntary urination and defecation.
- With syncope the animal is usually relaxed and almost always so at the *start* of the event. In some cases the legs can gradually become stiff, or even opisthotonus can develop. Urination sometimes occurs.

Level of consciousness
- In seizure activity, the animal is usually unconscious
- With cardiac syncope the animal can appear 'dazed' or unconscious, with a pre-syncopal event it is usually conscious
- With metabolic/endocrine disorders, the level of consciousness is variable
- With neuromuscular disorders, the animals are often fully conscious

Duration of episode
- A syncopal event usually last only seconds but occasionally minutes
- Seizures tend to last up to several minutes
- Metabolic/endocrine disorders tend to

produce confusion and a slow recovery over hours

Clinical observations
- Mucous membrane pallor often suggests a cardiac cause
- Cyanosis often suggests a respiratory disease or seizure activity
- A pronounced bradycardia (noticed by the owner on palpation of the cardiac area) may suggest a bradydysrhythmia
- Tachycardia may suggest a tachydysrhythmia or seizure, but could be associated with stress/fear on recovery

Recovery phase
- Following seizures, there is usually a recognisable post-ictal phase, in which the animal remains depressed/excited, sleepy/overactive, thirsty or hungry for minutes or, in extreme cases, for days after recovery
- Following a syncopal event recovery is rapid and complete with almost instant return to normality
- Recovery from a metabolic/endocrine cause can be prolonged and protracted and incomplete without medical intervention

CLINICAL EXAMINATION

- Often normal at the time of presentation, due to episodic nature of the collapsing, but a neurological examination can sometimes provide subtle clues.
- Examine thoroughly for evidence of *pain* associated with orthopaedic/spinal disease.
- If the collapse occurs following exercise then it is often worthwhile exercising the dog with the owner so that the reported symptoms can be witnessed and provide the opportunity for examination of colour and heart rate (+/– ECG event recording) during an episode.

CARDIORESPIRATORY SYNDROMES

OWNER EXAMINATION DURING THE COLLAPSE

- It might be practical to teach the owner how to examine the colour of the gums (they usually go pale with cardiac syncope) and feel the heart rate during future collapses (for an extreme bradycardia or tachycardia). It is, of course, important to have the owners practice daily so that they become familiar with what is normal.
- The information obtained from an owner can be misleading, and care should be taken in interpretation of such information.
- Another useful option is for the owner to record the event (camcorder, mobile videophone), particularly when the description of the event is unclear.

LABORATORY TESTS

- The blood sample must be taken from a fasted animal (e.g. 18 hours)
- The serum sample should be separated, especially those to be posted
- Haematology (including fresh, air-dried blood smears)
- Comprehensive biochemistry profile, with electrolytes
- Bile acids stimulation test – to screen for hepatic shunts
- Additional tests when indicated
  - Total T4 and TSH assay
  - ACTH stimulation test
  - Insulin assay (glucose:insulin ratio)
  - Acetylcholine receptor antibody (myasthenia gravis)
  - Faecal analysis for lungworm larvae
  - Heartworm testing (in enzootic areas)
  - Serum tests for *neospora, toxoplasma*

Haemorrhagic shock

Note: If occult haemorrhage is suspected, serial protein levels and haematology (including a reticulocyte count) should be run.

- PCV drops 12–24 hours after the haemorrhage
- Regenerative signs occur after four days and are maximal at seven days
- Protein levels drop after a few hours, up to 24 hours
- Check urine for evidence of blood breakdown products
- Ultrasound is the diagnostic test of choice to screen for abdominal fluid and for guided paracentesis

LONG ECG RHYTHM STRIP

- Arrhythmias that are present at the time of examination should be immediately apparent
- Even when the collapse is due to an arrhythmia, the ECG can be normal due to the arrhythmia's intermittent nature

AMBULATORY ECG RECORDING

- The identification of an arrhythmia causing collapse may only be possible with an ambulatory ECG machine
  - ECG event recorder
  - 24-hour Holter recorder
  - Implantable loop recorder (Reveal)
- For ambulatory monitoring to be effective, the animal must be collapsing regularly (at least once in 24 hours) or it must be possible to induce the collapse (e.g. by exercise)

RADIOGRAPHY

- Thoracic radiographs are of value in screening for heart or lung disease and thoracic masses
- The need for radiographs of the abdomen or skeletal system would be indicated by clinical examination

ULTRASOUND EXAMINATION

Ultrasound examination is of value in examining for heart diseases, occult abdominal haemorrhage or hepatic shunts.

ADDITIONAL TESTS

- Specialist neurological tests may be required and include electroencephalography (EEG) for CNS abnormalities, nerve conduction tests and electromyography (EMG) for peripheral neuropathies.
- Nerve/muscle biopsy.
- Response to *edrophonium chloride* can be used to test for myasthenia gravis. A dose of 0.11–0.22 mg/kg (to a maximum of 5 mg/dog) (slowly i/v) following fatigue/collapse on exercise usually produces an immediate and dramatic improvement with the effect lasting several minutes.

9 COUGH, DYSPNOEA AND TACHYPNOEA

COUGH

> **Cough:** A protective mechanism that involves a deep inspiration, followed by forced expiration against a closed glottis, with sudden opening of the glottis allowing expulsion of air at high velocity, bringing with it secretions that have accumulated in the larger airways.

FUNCTION OF THE COUGH REFLEX

The cough reflex is a mechanism that contributes to clearing the lung and airways of unwanted material and acts to expel inappropriate inhaled material. In combination with the mucociliary escalator and macrophage function at the level of the distal bronchioles and alveoli, coughing keeps the respiratory system clean. In certain disease situations coughing becomes more apparent, more frequent and more forceful. In certain diseases it is beneficial, while in others it is of little benefit to the patient.

STIMULI OF COUGHING

- Normal animals
  - Airway mucus
  - Small quantities of material inhaled during eating, drinking and breathing
- Diseased animals
  - Excessive airway mucus and other secretions
  - Excessive quantities of foreign material
  - Noxious irritants
  - Airway inflammation
  - Airway compression

TYPES OF COUGH

The type of cough may give some useful information but should not be relied upon to make a diagnosis.
- Harsh, hacking or dry cough
  - Diseases of larger airway
- Honking or 'seal-bark' cough
  - Tracheal collapse
  - Inhaled foreign bodies
- Soft, ineffectual cough
  - Diseases of the lower airways and lung parenchyma
- Exercise or nocturnal cough
  - Rarely assists diagnosis
  - Most animals will cough more during exercise or at night
- Productive cough
  - Animals rarely expectorate material or usually swallow expectorate material, so this is not often seen by the owner
  - Dogs often expectorate oropharyngeal material (i.e. saliva) at the end of a coughing episode
  - Haemoptysis may occur with neoplasia, foreign bodies, coagulopathies

DIFFERENTIAL DIAGNOSIS OF COUGHING

For causes of coughing see Table 9.1.

Clinical history

The factors to consider in the clinical history are:

- Age: Infectious diseases in youngsters, neoplasia in older animals
- Breed: Tracheal collapse in toy breeds, chronic bronchitis in terriers (see also Causes of congestive heart failure, Chapter 4)
- Possible exposure to an aetiological agent (infections, toxins etc.)

- Clinical signs attributable to other body systems (particularly gastrointestinal)
  - Vomiting or regurgitating
  - Pyrexia, lethargy
  - Anorexia, inappetance or cachexia
- Prior events
  - Surgery, trauma
- Response to therapy
- Presence of other cardiorespiratory signs
  - Exercise intolerance
  - Tachypnoea and dyspnoea
  - Collapse and syncope
  - Cyanosis
  - Ascites

Table 9.1 Conditions causing coughing (unlikely or rare causes are in parentheses)

Site	Condition
Upper Airway	(Tonsillitis)
	(Pharynx and larynx inflammation)
	(Neoplasia)
Trachea and Lower Airway	Tracheal collapse
	Extra-mural compression of trachea
	Acute tracheobronchitis
	Chronic tracheobronchial syndrome
	Chronic bronchitis
	Bronchiectasis
	Bronchial neoplasia
	Oslerus osleri
	Airway foreign bodies
	Feline asthma syndrome
Cardiac Disease	Left atrial enlargement
	Gross cardiomegaly
	Pulmonary oedema
Mediastinal Disease	Neoplasia (lymphosarcoma)
	Infections (nocardiosis)
Lung Parenchymal Disease	Pneumonia
	Viral and bacterial infections
	Aspiration pneumonia
	Pulmonary infiltration with eosinophilia
	Idiopathic pulmonary fibrosis
	Pulmonary abscesses
	Intrapulmonary haemorrhage
	Pulmonary neoplasia

CARDIORESPIRATORY SYNDROMES

Physical examination

The general physical examination of the cardiopulmonary patient is covered in detail in other sections and includes both the general physical examination and specific examination of the cardiac and respiratory systems.

DIAGNOSTIC TECHNIQUES

These are again covered in detail in other sections and include thoracic radiography, electrocardiography, cardiac ultrasound, bronchoscopy, biopsy techniques, blood gas analysis and haematology and blood biochemistry profiles.

> **Note:** Coughing with heart disease is usually due to compression of the mainstem bronchi by the enlarged heart, particularly an enlarged left atrium, and so tracheal elevation should be evident on a lateral chest X-ray.

TREATMENT

- As a rule, a productive cough is a necessary defence mechanism and should not be suppressed
- However, with non-productive coughs, including cardiac coughing, these can be suppressed

Cough suppressants

- Codeine linctus or tablets at 1–2 mg/kg q6–8h
- Butorphanol – 0.5–1.0 mg/kg i/m or s/c or q6–12h po

DIFFERENTIAL CLINICAL FEATURES OF SPECIFIC RESPIRATORY DISEASES

These diseases are discussed in more detail in the relevant sections of this book, and only a few points on these diseases and their association with coughing are included here. For cardiac causes of coughing see relevant sections.

Oropharynx

Pharyngitis, tonsillitis, laryngitis, etc. typically cause retching and choking rather than coughing.

Trachea

- *Tracheal collapse* – harsh honking cough
- *Acute tracheobronchitis* – dry and harsh cough
- *Chronic tracheobronchial syndrome/ tracheobronchitis* – mild paroxysmal harsh cough

Bronchi

- *Chronic bronchitis* – cough as an important protective mechanism
- *Bronchiectasis* – usually a sequel to chronic bronchitis
- *Inhaled foreign bodies* – very severe cough, becoming quieter as becomes chronic
- *Respiratory parasites* – will cause coughing

Distal airways and lung parenchyma

- *Pulmonary infiltration with eosinophilia (PIE)* – typically causes coughing
- *Feline asthma* – most common cause of cough in cats
- *Pneumonia* – cough is usually soft and ineffectual
- *Pulmonary haemorrhage* – similar to pneumonia, but animals are rarely pyrexic
- *Pulmonary neoplasia* – cough due to bronchial compression
- *Idiopathic pulmonary fibrosis* – cough in latter stages of the disease
- *Smoke inhalation* – evidence of having been in a house fire

SECTION 2

DYSPNOEA AND TACHYPNOEA

Dyspnoea and tachypnoea are common clinical presentations in cardiorespiratory disease, and indicate a significant degree of disease and respiratory impairment.

DEFINITIONS AND TERMINOLOGY

- Tachypnoea
  - Refers to an increased respiratory rate
  - Should not be confused with panting
- Dyspnoea
  - Laboured or difficult breathing
  - Best recognised when breathing is slow and purposeful
  - Inspiratory dyspnoea
    - Upper airway obstruction (stridor or stertor)
  - Expiratory dyspnoea
    - Discrete end-expiratory effort or grunt
    - Might only be heard on auscultation
    - Abdominal effort may be apparent
- Hyperpnoea
  - Deep and rapid breathing
    - Can be seen with hypoxic/cyanotic conditions without lung disease, e.g. right-to-left cardiac shunts
- Orthopnoea (severe and life-threatening)
  - Adopting a standing or sternal position to ease breathing. Typically noted as:
    - Cats – sternal recumbency, abducted elbows, extended neck, open-mouthed breathing
    - Dogs – remaining standing, reluctance to lie down

DIFFERENTIAL DIAGNOSIS

For a list of conditions causing dyspnoea, see Table 9.2.

Clinical history

The features of the clinical history relevant to the differential diagnosis of dyspnoea and tachypnoea are similar to those for coughing.

PHYSICAL EXAMINATION

The physical examination is similar to that for the whole respiratory system and is covered in detail in other sections. However, with respect to dyspnoea and tachypnoea, care often has to be taken when examining the patient so as not to precipitate a respiratory crisis. Also, observation of the breathing pattern may have to take place once the patient is hospitalised and in a quiet, undisturbed environment. Additionally, attention must be paid to the extrathoracic airways.

Extrathoracic airways and causes of dyspnoea and tachypnoea

- Examine closely from the nares to the thoracic inlet
- Check for presence of nasal discharges
- Check conformity of the head, and integrity of the larynx and trachea
- Identify if there is fever or heat stroke and if the animal has been exercising or is excited
- Check for abdominal distension, obesity, anaemia, evidence of metabolic acidosis and neurological disorders

LOCALISATION OF SOURCE AND CAUSE OF RESPIRATORY DISTRESS

- Upper airway obstruction can be identified on auscultation
  - Inspiratory stridor or stertor

CARDIORESPIRATORY SYNDROMES

Table 9.2 Conditions causing dyspnoea (unlikely or rare causes are in parentheses)

Site	Condition
Upper Airway	Stenotic nares
	Rhinitis
	Nasal neoplasia
	Brachycephalic airway syndrome
	Extended soft palate
	Laryngeal paralysis
	Laryngeal collapse
Trachea and Lower Airway	Tracheal collapse
	Hypoplastic trachea
	(Tracheal stenosis)
	Extra-mural compression of trachea
	Chronic bronchitis
	Bronchiectasis
	(Bronchial neoplasia)
	Airway foreign bodies
	Feline asthma syndrome
Cardiac Disease	Pulmonary oedema
	Pleural effusion
Mediastinal Disease	Neoplasia
	Infections
Lung Parenchymal Disease	Bronchopneumonia
	Aspiration pneumonia
	Pulmonary infiltration with eosinophilia
	Non-cardiogenic pulmonary oedema
	Idiopathic pulmonary fibrosis
	Intrapulmonary haemorrhage
	Pulmonary neoplasia
Pleural Disease/Thoracic Damage	Pleural effusion
	Ruptured diaphragm
	Fractured rib(s)

- ○ Nasal, pharyngeal, laryngeal and tracheal disease
- Inspiratory crackles
  - ○ Restrictive lung disease (pulmonary oedema, pulmonary fibrosis)
- End-expiratory dyspnoea
  - ○ Non-fixed airway obstruction
  - ○ Intrathoracic tracheal collapse
- ○ Neoplasms
- ○ Feline asthma (lung hyperinflation)
- Combination of inspiratory dyspnoea, expiratory dyspnoea and wheezing
  - ○ Fixed airway obstructions
  - ○ Bronchoconstriction (feline asthma)
  - ○ Intraluminal masses (rare)
- Tachypnoea without dyspnoea

- ○ Restriction of lung expansion
  Lung parenchymal diseases (pneumonia)
  Pleural effusions
  Chest restriction (abdominal, diaphragmatic, neuromuscular and chest-wall abnormalities)
- ○ Non-respiratory conditions (fever, shock, anaemia and acidosis)

> **Note:** It is often very difficult to identify the actual cause of dyspnoea and tachypnoea on physical examination or by assessing the nature of the abnormal breathing pattern.

DIAGNOSTIC TECHNIQUES

These are again covered in detail in other sections, and include thoracic radiography, electrocardiography, cardiac ultrasound, bronchoscopy, biopsy techniques, blood gas analysis, haematology and blood biochemistry.

DIFFERENTIAL CLINICAL FEATURES OF SPECIFIC RESPIRATORY DISEASES

These diseases are discussed in more detail in the relevant sections of this book, and only a few points on them and their association with dyspnoea are included here. For cardiac causes of dyspnoea see relevant sections.

Nasal
Rhinitis and *neoplasia* will cause stertor if there is sufficient nasal obstruction.

Oropharynx
Brachycephalic airway syndrome, hypoplastic trachea, extended soft palate, laryngeal paralysis will invariably cause dyspnoea.

Trachea
- *Tracheal collapse* – Usually causes cough, but will cause dyspnoea if severe
- *Hypoplastic trachea* (see brachycephalic airway syndrome, pp. 000–000)

Bronchi
- *Chronic bronchitis* – Dyspnoea if very severe or causing secondary lung changes
- *Bronchiectasis* – see Chronic bronchitis, pp. 151–2
- *Inhaled foreign bodies* – Dyspnoea, only if there is severe airway obstruction, usually rostral to the carina

Distal airways and lung parenchyma
- *Pulmonary infiltration with eosinophilia (PIE)* – Coughing mainly, except if extensive and severe disease (rare)
- *Feline asthma* – Common cause of dyspnoea (usually paroxysmal) in cats
- *Pneumonia* – Dyspnoea, when disease is severe
- *Pulmonary haemorrhage* – As for pneumonia
- *Pulmonary neoplasia* – Towards the terminal stages of the disease, when disease is extensive; when compressing a large airway (audible expiratory dyspnoea)
- *Idiopathic pulmonary fibrosis* – Dyspnoea with advanced disease, but usually the first thing noticed by the owner, along with exercise intolerance

CARDIORESPIRATORY SYNDROMES

SECTION 3

DISEASES OF THE CARDIORESPIRATORY SYSTEM

10 DISEASES OF THE VALVES AND ENDOCARDIUM

- Diseases of the valves may be congenital or acquired. A list of the primary diseases of the endocardium and valves is given in Table 10.1.
- Any disease affecting any part of the mitral valve complex may result in poor coaptation of the valve cusps and thus incompetence (insufficiency), with regurgitation of blood into the left atrium from the ventricle. Mitral regurgitation itself will lead to left atrial dilation and widening of the valve annulus.

Eventually congestive heart failure may occur.
- Congenital lesions affecting the cardiac valves are discussed in Chapter 13. Acquired mitral valve disease is the most common heart disease in the dog, but is rare in the cat. Valvular insufficiency (functional regurgitation) may occur secondary to other cardiac diseases such as dilated cardiomyopathy or congenital shunts, and this is discussed in the relevant sections.

Table 10.1 A summary of the more common primary diseases of the cardiac valves

Valve	Primary Diseases	Congenital or Acquired	Incidence
Mitral	Endocardiosis	Acquired	Common
	Endocarditis	Acquired	Rare
	Dysplasia	Congenital	Uncommon
Tricuspid	Endocardiosis	Acquired	Relatively common
	Endocarditis	Acquired	Very rare
	Dysplasia	Congenital	Uncommon
Aortic	Endocarditis	Acquired	Uncommon
	Stenosis	Congenital	Common
Pulmonic	Stenosis	Congenital	Relatively common

MITRAL VALVE DISEASE (MVD)

Also referred to as *myxomatous mitral valve disease* or *mitral valve endocardiosis*, mitral valve disease is the most common heart disease leading to left-sided conges-

tive failure in adult dogs. It is uncommon in the cat, and most common in small- to medium-sized breeds of dog. The disease has a strong age association, and all geriatric dogs probably have some pathological evidence of the disease, although many are clinically unaffected. Males are more commonly affected than females (1.5:1), and 30% of cases will also have tricuspid involvement.

BREEDS OF DOG COMMONLY AFFECTED WITH MITRAL VALVE DISEASE

- Cavalier King Charles Spaniel
- Poodle
- Schnauzer
- Chihuahua
- Fox Terrier
- Boston Terrier

AETIOLOGY

The aetiology is unknown at present, although there may be an hereditary component in view of the prevalence in some breeds.

PATHOPHYSIOLOGY

Mitral regurgitation progresses, leading to:
- Volume loading of the left atrium and then also the left ventricle
- Increase in both the preload and afterload on the heart
- Forward failure (reduced cardiac output)
- Left ventricular and atrial dilation leading to dilation of the valve annulus and further regurgitation
- Pulmonary congestion with the usual signs of left-sided congestive failure
- In long standing cases, left ventricular myocardial failure eventually develops
- Rupture of a *chordae tendineae* may occur, resulting in rapid onset of left-sided congestive failure (1–2 hours)

CLINICAL FINDINGS

- Clinical signs develop in middle aged or older dogs
- Systolic murmur is noted prior to the signs of heart failure
  - Heard maximally over the apex of the heart
  - Initially protosystolic and soft, but progresses to pansystolic
  - Can radiate widely on the left, to the right and along the trachea
  - A loud *whooping* musical systolic murmur with a palpable thrill is often characteristic of a prolapsed mitral valve
- A mid-systolic click is occasionally heard early in the course of the disease
- In more advanced disease an S3 gallop sound can sometimes be appreciated, occurring just after the murmur (can be mistaken for S2)
- Cough
  - Left atrial enlargement compressing the left mainstem bronchus
  - The cough may be nocturnal, noticed early in the morning and associated with excitement or lead pulling
- Heart failure
  - Chronic and slowly progressive, but acute decompensation can occur
  - Eventual left-sided congestive heart failure (Chapter 6)
    - Dyspnoea and tachypnoea
  - Right-sided congestive failure may also be present if there is also tricuspid valve endocardiosis
  - Rupture of a *chordae tendineae* presents as an acute and unexpected onset of left-sided congestive heart failure
- Syncope is sometimes seen (cause unknown)
  - Vasovagal effect
  - Supraventricular tachycardia
  - Tussive syncope
- The findings on physical examination are usually typical of those for congestive heart failure (Chapter 6)

DIAGNOSIS

Clinical features

Classical clinical presentation is very useful in diagnosis of MVD.

Clinical pathology

- Prerenal azotaemia is common with moderate to severe heart failure
- ProANP is usually elevated when there is significant left or right atrial dilation
- Raised liver enzymes – when there is right-sided congestive failure

Electrocardiography

- Left atrial (prolonged P waves) and ventricular enlargement pattern (tall and prolonged QRS complexes) may be seen
- Rhythm can vary from normal sinus arrhythmia to a compensatory sinus tachycardia, supraventricular premature complexes, supraventricular tachycardia or atrial fibrillation
- Ventricular premature complexes or ventricular tachycardia are uncommon

Radiography

Radiography is important in diagnosis and for identification of left atrial enlargement and assessment of the severity of pulmonary oedema. It is useful as well for screening for airway diseases which are also common in small breed dogs.

- Radiography is sensitive for detecting left atrial enlargement. On lateral views, this can vary from a mild straightening of the caudal border of the heart (loss of the caudal cardiac waist) to massive bulging of the left atrium caudodorsally causing marked dorsal displacement of the distal trachea and mainstem bronchi.
- Splitting of the mainstem bronchi and compression of the left bronchus may be seen on lateral views.
- In advanced cases, generalised cardiomegaly develops.

> **Note:** Coughing, with heart disease, is usually due to compression of the mainstem bronchi by the enlarged heart, particularly an enlarged left atrium (tracheal elevation should be evident on a lateral chest X-ray). As a guideline, if the cough is associated with cardiomegaly the vertebral heart score typically exceeds 11.5 (and length >6.5).

Signs of left-sided congestive failure

- Enlargement of the pulmonary veins
- Interstitial to alveolar pulmonary oedema, often more marked in the perihilar region

Signs of right-sided congestive heart failure

- Enlargement of the caudal vena cava
- Pleural effusion
- Hepatomegaly and ascites

Echocardiography

- Left atrium dilatation of varying degrees
- Left ventricular dilation also develops in more severe cases
- Left ventricular contractility is good in early stage MVD; can appear hyperdynamic where there is a volume overload (Frank-Starling mechanism)
- Left ventricular failure develops in time

> **Note:** In dogs with a normal fractional shortening, those with severe regurgitation and cardiac enlargement are likely to have myocardial failure.

- Variable degree of nodular thickening on valve cusps
- Regurgitant flow identifiable on Doppler echocardiography (colour and spectral)
- Rupture of the *chordae tendineae* causing flail leaflet (cusp) (uncommon)
- Left atrial tear (uncommon)

THERAPY

- Treatment is not indicated if the patient is asymptomatic (murmur only). When symptomatic, treatment is aimed at the signs of heart failure (see Chapter 6, p. 68).
- As the disease progresses, therapy is required to assist in maintaining compensation, with increasing doses and additional drugs to maintain a satisfactory quality of life.
- The availability of surgical treatment (valve repair or replacement) is very limited.

Main drugs used in the treatment of mitral valve disease
- ACE inhibitors
- Furosemide – minimum effective dose
- Digoxin – for atrial fibrillation
- Pimobendan
- Antitussive drugs

ACE inhibitors
- Enalapril, ramipril, benazepril, imidapril
  - In advanced and long-standing heart failure, the dose can be doubled to twice daily

Furosemide
- When there is radiographic evidence of congestion/oedema
- Dose proportional to the severity of congestion/oedema
- Dose range is 1–4 mg/kg bid, but typical starting dose, with mild to moderate congestion, is 1–2 mg/kg

Inotropic agents
- Indicated when myocardial failure develops, but there is some debate about the benefit of inotropic agents in early stage MVD
  - Pimobendan

Digoxin
- For the control of supraventricular tachydysrhythmias, particularly atrial fibrillation (for dose see Chapter 6, Table 6.2, p. 69)
- Measurement of serum digoxin levels is recommended to ensure correct dosing

β-blockers and calcium channel blockers
- Alternative options for the control of supraventricular tachyarrhythmias
- These are negative inotropic drugs and should be used with caution

Exercise restriction
- Essential when the dog is in congestive failure
- Limited exercise once the congestive failure is controlled

Treatment of acute fulminant pulmonary oedema (see p. 66)
- Strict rest
- Sedation to relieve anxiety – morphine, diazepam, butorphanol
- Furosemide (3–4 mg/kg every two hours initially), administered i/v, (if restraint is not stressful), otherwise i/m
- Percutaneous glyceryl trinitrate – 0.5–5 cm tid (depending on the size of dog)
- Supplemental oxygen, without any form of restraint
- Pimobendan orally or i/v dobutamine and sodium nitroprusside

Coughing
- Chronic coughing is a common problem.
- The primary cause of the cough is due to compression of the left mainstem bronchus by the enlarged left atrium.
- The aim of therapy is to reduce the frequency/severity of coughing to an acceptable level.
- Adequate control of congestion is the first priority, but it is also important to avoid over-diuresis.

- Antitussive drugs are indicated to suppress the non-productive coughing associated with cardiomegaly:
  - Codeine 0.5–2.0 mg/kg q8–12h po
  - Butorphanol 0.5–1.0 mg/kg i/m or s/c or q6–12h po
- An occasional injection of a non-steroidal anti-inflammatory drug may also be used to help reduce airway inflammation secondary to the airway compression and coughing.
- Coughing may also be associated with oedema fluid flooding the airways (alveolar oedema), however this is a less common cause. This is associated with advanced or acute left-sided congestive failure and should be recognised by the dog coughing up a pink-tinged frothy fluid. Should this happen, immediate and urgent treatment is necessary (see Chapter 6, p. 66).

PROGNOSIS

In the early stages of MVD the cardiovascular system is able to compensate satisfactorily for many years. Once signs of heart failure develop, the prognosis is less predictable. Dogs in which coughing associated with cardiomegaly is the primary problem, often seem to survive for a few years, but, once pulmonary oedema develops, survival is often less than a year. Possible adverse outcomes include rupture of chordae tendineae, left atrial rupture and tachydysrhythmias. Ultimately, therapy will be unable to maintain cardiac compensation and congestive failure will progress, with the necessity for euthanasia.

SECONDARY MITRAL VALVE INCOMPETENCE

- This occurs as a result of dilation of the mitral valve annulus due to left atrial and/or ventricular dilation, such as in dilated cardiomyopathy.
- Large congenital (left-to-right) shunts (e.g. PDA, VSD) result in supranormal volumes being diverted through the pulmonary circulation, which, on return to the left heart, lead to left atrial dilation and mitral valve incompetence.
- Cardiomyopathy in cats may lead to distortion of the mitral valve apparatus, poor coaptation of the valve cusps, and thus valvular incompetence.

TRICUSPID VALVE ENDOCARDIOSIS

- The tricuspid valve is rarely affected by endocardiosis alone (<2% of cases) but is seen more commonly in conjunction with mitral valve disease. Approximately a third of dogs with endocardiosis will have lesions on both mitral and tricuspid valves.
- The main difference from mitral valve disease is therefore the involvement of the right side of the heart and thus the development of right-sided congestive failure. The treatment is similar, although a greater level of diuresis may be required when right-sided congestive failure is present.

DISEASES OF THE CARDIORESPIRATORY SYSTEM

VALVULAR ENDOCARDITIS

Also referred to as infective or bacterial endocarditis, this is a rare disease that may be over diagnosed. The valves are the most common location for infection, but the mural endocardium, septal defects and patent ductus arteriosus can become infected. Reported in medium- to large-breed dogs, with the German Shepherd and Boxer predominating. It is more common in dogs older than four years of age.

AETIOLOGY AND PATHOPHYSIOLOGY

- Bacteraemia is the likely source of cardiac infection
  - Periodontal disease
  - Gastrointestinal or urogenital tract, prostate, skin, bone or lung infections
  - Can also be iatrogenic (intravenous catheterisation)
  - Gram negative or Gram positive aerobes; anaerobes are rare
  - *Staphylococcus* spp, *Escherichia coli*, *Erysipelothrix rhusiopathiae*, *Streptococcus* spp, *Corynebacterium* spp, and *Pseudomonas aeruginosa*
- Vegetative thrombi of varying size and shape
- Aortic valve affected in 90% of cases, but the mitral valve can also be affected
- Systemic embolisation can lead to infarction and/or metastatic infection
  - Kidneys and spleen, but other sites include: brain, intestine and coronary arteries

CLINICAL FINDINGS

Systemic signs
Systemic signs of persistent or recurrent infection:

- Weakness, lethargy, lameness, anorexia and weight loss
- Shifting-leg lameness (septic or immune-mediated arthritis)
- Retinal haemorrhage, petechiation, hyphaema, epistaxis, cold or cyanotic extremities and joint pain or stiffness
- Animals can develop septic shock, which often leads to death

Cardiac signs
- A new murmur, or one that changes its character, or a murmur of aortic regurgitation (left base, diastolic) with a hyperkinetic pulse
- Valvular incompetence (aortic and mitral) incompetence leading to left-sided congestive failure

DIAGNOSIS

Laboratory diagnosis
- Blood culture of the causative bacteria
  - Two to three samples (10–20 ml blood per sample) within a 24-hour period, preferably during periods of pyrexia
- Specific culture bottles containing appropriate medium are required
- Submit for aerobic and anaerobic culture
- Important bacteria can be cultured in seven days; may take three weeks
- An organism is considered significant if it is cultured from at least two samples
- 50–75% positive blood culture with bacterial endocarditis in dogs
- Negative culture may be obtained

Electrocardiography
- Variable; may show chamber-enlargement pattern
- Dysrhythmias and conduction defects in 75% of cases
- Severe arrhythmias may be associated with a poorer prognosis

Radiography
- Changes non-specific, but may show the presence of congestive failure and/or chamber enlargement

Echocardiography
Important in the visualisation of vegetative lesions on the aortic or mitral valves:
- Two-dimensional echocardiography can detect vegetative lesions as a small as 2 mm
- Lesions on the aortic valve are virtually pathognomonic, whereas those on the mitral valve are difficult to distinguish from endocardiosis
- Serial echocardiographic examinations are useful to check for morphologic changes in subtle lesions where the diagnosis might be uncertain
- Endocarditis results in valvular incompetence

THERAPY

- Therapy is aimed at:
  - Eliminating the infection
  - Management of any systemic signs
  - Management of heart failure
  - Control of arrhythmias

- Antibiotic selection on the basis of culture and sensitivity *in vitro*
  - Empirical while awaiting bacterial culture results
    - bactericidal antibiotics active against Gram positive and Gram negative aerobes
    - Anti-anaerobes may be needed
    - Penicillins, fluoroquinolones, metronidazole, clindamycin
- Initially given parenterally (ideally intravenously) to ensure therapeutic concentrations are achieved, followed by at least six weeks of oral medication
- Important to treat extracardiac infection
- Treatment of congestive heart failure (Chapter 6) and arrhythmias (Chapter 7) if symptomatic

PROGNOSIS

Prognosis is guarded to poor, with many cases dying from congestive heart failure, arrhythmias, sepsis or renal failure. Survival time varies from days to two years, but the majority usually die or are euthanased within a few months of diagnosis.

11 DISEASES OF THE MYOCARDIUM

CARDIOMYOPATHY

The term cardiomyopathy refers to conditions that primarily affect the heart muscle in the absence of inflammation and with no identifiable congenital or acquired disease. Different cardiomyopathies have different prevalances in dogs and cats (see Table 11.1).

TABLE 11.1 Prevalence of cardiomyopathies in the dog and cat compared

Disease	Prevalence in Dogs	Prevalence in Cats
Dilated Cardiomyopathy	The most common form of cardiomyopathy in dogs	Very rare
Hypertrophic Cardiomyopathy	Very rare	Probably accounts for $2/3$ of the adult heart disease
Arrhythmogenic Right Ventricular Cardiomyopathy (ARVC)	Uncommon – the Boxer dog is the most commonly affected breed	Very rare
Tachycardia-induced Myocardial Failure	Uncommon	n/a
Restrictive Cardiomyopathy	n/a	Probably accounts for $1/4$ of adult heart disease

DILATED CARDIOMYOPATHY (DCM)

Dilated cardiomyopathy can be:
- Primary (idiopathic)
  - Hypocontractile and dilated left ventricle, with no identifiable cause
- Secondary
  - Taurine deficiency
  - L-carnitine deficiency
  - Tachycardia-induced failure
  - Toxic factors, e.g. doxorubicin
- DCM is more commonly seen in medium- to large-breed dogs; rarely seen in small-breed dogs weighing less than 15 kg
- More common in male
- Mean age at presentation is 6–7 years old (range 0.5–14 years)
- More than 90% of dogs are pure bred; rare in mixed-breed dogs
- It is rare in cats since commercial cat food has been supplemented with taurine, but was formerly seen more commonly in middle-aged Siamese, Burmese and Abyssinian breeds, in both sexes.

BREEDS AFFECTED BY IDIOPATHIC DCM

- Dobermann
- Boxer
- Great Dane
- Cocker Spaniel
- German Shepheard Dog
- Saint Bernard
- Labrador
- Irish Wolfhound
- Golden Retriever
- Newfoundland

AETIOLOGY

- Unknown, but may involve a genetic biochemical defect, prior viral infection (e.g. enterovirus), immunological abnormalities and chemical toxins
- Familial predisposition in several breeds including the Dobermann, Boxer and Cocker Spaniel
- Secondary causes, such as taurine deficiency in the cat, doxorubicin toxicity and L-carnitine deficiency in the dog

PATHOPHYSIOLOGY

- Myocardium unable to generate the pressures required to maintain cardiac output (systolic failure)
- Ventricles become stretched and volume overloaded
- The ventricles become non-compliant, failing to relax, compromising ventricular filling (diastolic failure)
- Atrioventricular (AV) rings become stretched allowing regurgitation of blood into the atria
- Atrial pressures increase, the atria become dilated, pressures in the veins behind the heart increase, leading to congestive heart failure (see Chapter 6)

CLINICAL FEATURES

- May have a long sub-clinical (asymptomatic) course (occult DCM) – 2–4 years in Dobermanns
- Short clinical history (days to weeks)

Presenting signs

- Breathlessness
- Cough
- Weakness
- Exercise intolerance
- Inappetance
- Collapse – a common presentation in Boxers
- Lethargy
- Weight loss
- Sudden death

Common clinical findings

- Weak pulse
- Tachycardia
- Pale mucous membranes and cold extremities (poor peripheral perfusion)
- Cough (cardiomegaly causing airway compression and/or alveolar oedema)
- S3 gallop sound on auscultation
- Murmurs of mitral and/or tricuspid regurgitation, but they can be very quiet (grade 1–3) and difficult to appreciate, particularly if there is an arrhythmia, such as atrial fibrillation
- Dyspnoea and tachypnoea – due to pulmonary oedema
- Right-heart failure signs
  - Distended jugular veins
  - Hepatomegaly
  - Ascites
  - Percussable pleural fluid line
- Pleural effusion is more common in cats, which can be:
  - Chylous
  - Modified transudate

DIAGNOSIS

Clinical pathology

- Pre-renal azotaemia – urea increased more than creatinine
- Liver enzymes can be elevated due to hepatic congestion
- Mild decrease in protein levels
- Mild decrease in sodium
- ProANP and troponin may be elevated

Electrocardiography

- The ECG often demonstrates left ventricular and atrial enlargement pattern
- Atrial fibrillation in giant-breed dogs (70–80%)
- Ventricular premature complexes are common, particularly in Dobermanns and Boxers (see Holter monitoring, below)
- In cats, sinus rhythm (50%) and bradycardias are common (25%)

Holter monitoring

24-hour ECG monitoring is increasingly available, and annual Holter recording can assist in making a diagnosis as well as monitoring rhythm disturbances.

- Boxers (also see Arrhythmogenic right ventricular cardiomyopathy)
  - Morphology of VPCs in Boxers often of right ventricular origin
- Dobermanns
  - Three quarters have VPCs or VT on a 24-hour Holter recording
  - >50 VPCs per 24-hour Holter is suggestive of occult DCM
  - Presence of a sustained (>30 secs) ventricular tachycardia is a predictor of sudden death

Radiography

Radiography is *not specific for DCM*, but findings may include:

- Left atrial enlargement, cardiomegaly with rounding of the cardiac apex and radiographic signs of congestive failure
- Pulmonary venous congestion

- Pulmonary oedema: often in the perihilar and/or dorsal caudal lung lobes; can sometimes seem denser in the right lung compared to the left
- Enlarged caudal vena cava
- Minimal cardiomegaly may be seen in Dobermanns and Boxers
- Pleural effusion tends to be a more common finding in congestive heart failure (CHF) in cats

Echocardiography

Echocardiography is required to make a diagnosis of DCM and define the extent of systolic dysfunction. The guidelines are shown below. The differentiation of DCM versus mitral valve disease in larger breed dogs can be difficult

- Demonstrates enlarged, dilated and rounded left ventricular chamber
- Measurements of left ventricular chamber size (systole and diastole) can be obtained from 2-D and M-mode tracing of the left ventricle (see Chapter 4)
- Poor left ventricular contractility is subjectively observed on the moving 2-D image Fractional shortening is an insensitive and non-specific indicator of DCM, but a FS% <15% would be considered suggestive of DCM

Criteria for diagnosis of classical DCM in dogs

- Increased left ventricular systolic diameter
- Globoid left ventricle
- Increased left ventricular diastolic diameter
- Decreased fractional shortening
  - 15–20% mild to moderately severe (should not have pulmonary oedema)
  - <15% severe (likely to have pulmonary oedema)
- Increased E point to septal separation (EPSS): >7 mm
- Left atrium is dilated but not dis-

TABLE 11.2 Criteria for the diagnosis of dilated cardiomyopathy in selected breeds of dog

Breed	Condition	Parameter	Diagnostic Value	Mean (SD)	Reference
Dobermann	Subclinical	LVDd (mm)	>46	No values	O'Grady
	DCM	LVDs (mm)	>38		& Horne
		FS (%)	<15		(1995)
Irish	Subclinical	LVDd (mm)	No values	60 (6.4)	Vollmar
Wolfhound	DCM	LVDs (mm)		42 (4.4)	(1999a)
		FS (%)		25 (4.5)	
	Clinical	LVDd (mm)	No values	67 (6.2)	
	DCM	LVDs (mm)		52 (8.0)	
		FS (%)		13.5 (3.6)	
Newfoundland	Clinical	LVDd (mm)	No values	51 (7.1)	Dukes-
	DCM	LVDs (mm)		43 (5.6)	McEwan
		FS (%)		15.7 (5.3)	(1999)

proportionately larger than the left ventricular diastolic diameter
- Decreased aortic outflow velocity
- Increased PEP:ET ratio (>0.75)
- Ejection fraction (measured by Simpson's rule) <40%

Criteria for diagnosis of DCM in cats
- Left ventricular systolic diameter >16 mm
- Rounded (globoid) ventricular chamber
- Increased E point to septal separation >4 mm
- Decreased systolic wall thickening

THERAPY

Treatment is aimed at controlling the signs of heart failure and providing positive inotropic support for the heart (see Chapter 6, p. 68).
- *ACE inhibitors*, with the dose being doubled as the disease progresses
- *Diuretics* are usually required, but the dose

must be proportional to the severity of congestion and then reduced when the congestion reduces, ensuring minimum effective levels are used
  - Furosemide, typically starting at 1–2 mg/kg q12h with mild to moderate congestion
- *Exercise restriction* is essential when the dog is in congestive failure; once controlled, exercise is recommended, but within the limits of ability for the dog
- *Inotropic agents* (e.g. pimobendan) are indicated to improve ventricular contractility (see p. 69)
- *Digoxin* to control atrial fibrillation (see p. 68)
- *Chronic and intractable ascites* is not uncommon with DCM. In these cases additional diuretics can be added (see p. 70) (furosemide dose usually not exceeding 4 mg/kg bid) – drug options are:
  - Co-amilozide (amiloride + hydrochlorothiazide)
  - Spironolactone
- *Ventricular arrhythmias* can be controlled with (see p. 73):
  - Mexilitine (5–8 mg/kg tid)
  - Sotalol (0.5–2 mg/kg bid)

DISEASES OF THE CARDIORESPIRATORY SYSTEM

Out-patient treatment of congestive heart failure due to DCM in dogs (see p. 68)

- Initial rest – until decompensated failure is controlled
- Furosemide 1–4 mg/kg bid – dose proportional to severity of oedema
- ACE inhibitor – initially at standard dose, but doubling to bid in progressive cases
- Digoxin – for control of atrial fibrillation
- Pimobendan – for inotropic support
- Add co-amilozide or spironolactone – for intractable ascites
- Anti-arrhythmics – if significant arrhythmias present

Treatment of acute fulminant pulmonary oedema due to DCM in dogs (see p. 66)

- Strict cage rest
- Oxygen supplementation – without any form of restraint (additional stress)
- Furosemide adminstered i/v (if restraint is not stressful), otherwise i/m (4 mg/kg every 1–2 hours until diuresis is evident and dyspnoea reduces)
- Percutaneous glyceryl trinitrate and oral pimobendan *or* Na nitroprusside at 1.0–10.0 μg/kg/min i/v + dobutamine at 5.0–10 μg/kg/min i/v

Additional therapy

Taurine supplementation

- Plasma taurine concentrations often low in Cocker Spaniels and Golden Retrievers
- Newfoundlands have often been found to have low blood taurine levels and should be supplemented with taurine
- The dose for taurine supplementation is 500 mg per dog bid

- Any cat with DCM (rare finding) should be supplemented with taurine, even if it has been fed a taurine replete diet, at a dose of 250 mg per cat bid; response on echocardiography should be noted in 3–4 months

L-carnitine supplementation

L-carnitine can be deficient in up to 50% of dogs with DCM, but identification of true deficiency is difficult and impractical. Supplementation at 50 mg/kg q8h might be worthwhile in Boxers, American Cocker Spaniels and Dobermanns. Response on echocardiography should be noted in 3–4 months.

Fish oil supplementation

- May improve appetite and be of benefit in controlling the cachexia commonly found with chronic congestive heart failure
  - It is proposed that this is as a result of reducing the elevated cytokine levels
- Recommended doses for supplementation:
  - Eicosapentaenoic acid (EPA) – 40 mg/kg per day
  - Docosahexaenoic acid (DHA) – 25 mg/kg per day

B vitamins

Due to loss through the urine in chronically diuresed dogs, B-vitamin supplementation should be considered.

PROGNOSIS

- Survival time for DCM is generally considered poor but is very breed dependent
  - 50% survival is 12 weeks, although the overall mean is eight months
  - Survival at one year is 20% and at two years is 5–10%
- Dobermanns, Labradors, German Shepherds and Great Danes often have a short survival time, whereas Cocker

Spaniels, Irish Wolfhounds and Golden Retrievers often have a longer survival time

- Sudden death, probably due to ventricular tachycardia leading to ventricular fibrillation, is more common in Dobermanns and Boxers

- 80% of dogs that are in atrial fibrillation will have died by six months from the time of diagnosis
- In the remainder, death or euthanasia results from continuing uncontrollable congestive heart failure and/or cachexia

ARRHYTHMOGENIC RIGHT VENTRICULAR CARDIOMYOPATHY (ARVC)

AETIOLOGY

- Fibro-fatty infiltration affecting primarily the right ventricular myocardium
- Primarily seen in Boxers, but also reported in other breeds
- Rare in the cat – but can easily be misdiagnosed as tricuspid valve dysplasia
- An inherited disorder, believed to be an autosomal dominant trait with incomplete penetrance

CLINICAL SIGNS

- Severe arrhythmias
- Asymptomatic
- Syncope
- Congestive heart failure
- Sudden death

DIAGNOSIS

Histopathology is required to make a definitive diagnosis in many cases.

ECG

- Marked ventricular arrhythmias of right ventricular origin (left bundle branch morphology)
- Holter monitoring is useful in the screening of suspected dogs, with >100 VPCs over 24 hours being suspicious (see also Table 11.3)

TABLE 11.3 Interpretation of 24-hour Holter monitoring in Boxers

Number of VPCs	Interpretation
<20	Normal
20–100	Indeterminate – repeat in 6–12 months
100–300	Suspicious
300–1000 or	Likely affected
100–300 with	Likely affected
couplets, triplets or VT	
>1000	Affected

Echocardiography

Echocardiography usually does not demonstrate any abnormality, although in some cases enlargement of the right ventricle may be present.

THERAPY

- Treatment of ventricular arrhythmias (see p. 73)
  - Sotalol: 0.5–2 mg/kg bid
  - Mexiletine: 5–8 mg/kg tid + low-dose atenolol 0.3–0.5 mg/kg bid
- Holter monitoring is useful for assessing response to treatment

TACHYCARDIA-INDUCED MYOCARDIAL FAILURE

Primarily seen in dogs following a period (days to weeks) of sustained high-rate tachycardia (>250/min), most commonly a supraventricular tachycardia (SVT).

PATHOPHYSIOLOGY

- The tachycardia results in reduced filling time, a reduced stroke volume and increased myocardial oxygen consumption
- Myocardial contractility decreases; on echocardiography can mimic dilated cardiomyopathy
- Leads to congestive heart failure

THERAPY

- Supportive treatment for the congestive heart failure is usually required
- If/when the tachyarrhythmia is controlled, the myocardial failure and congestive heart failure are usually reversible
- After cardioversion of the tachycardia, myocardial function can take weeks to recover

HYPERTROPHIC CARDIOMYOPATHY (HCM)

HCM is the single most common heart disease in cats. It is rare in the dog. The obstructive form is termed hypertrophic obstructive cardiomyopathy (HOCM) (see p. 110).

AETIOLOGY

- Unknown at this time, but thought to be a genetic defect, as it is in humans
- Pedigree breed predisposition is seen (Maine Coon) but it is also common in domestic short- and longhaired cats

CLINICAL FEATURES

- Mean age at presentation is 5–7 years (range 5 months to 14 years)
- The incidence is greater in male cats
- Many cats are asymptomatic
- HCM might only be diagnosed at post mortem following an unexpected death

Presenting signs

- Tachypnoea
- Dyspnoea due to peracute pulmonary oedema and/or pleural effusion
- Lethargy
- Inappetence
- Exercise intolerance
- Syncope – due to tachyarrhythmias or dynamic left ventricular outflow tract obstruction
- Thromboembolism (see this chapter, pp. 114–15)

Note: Coughing is very rare in cats with heart disease.

Clinical findings

- A hyperdynamic apex beat
- Gallop sound (often S4)
- Murmur (varies from grade 1–5) due to:
  - Dynamic outflow tract obstruction (murmur louder during periods of tachycardia and quieter when the cat relaxes and the heart rate reduces)
  - Mitral regurgitation (best heard at the left apex or on the sternum)

- Arrhythmias – premature beats with pulse deficit
- Pulmonary crackles due to airway oedema may be auscultated
- Pleural effusion may cause muffling of heart and lung sounds

DIAGNOSIS

Clinical pathology
- Pre-renal azotaemia
- Hypokalaemia – when anorexic
- Serum troponin I usually elevated

Electrocardiography
Electrocardiogrpahy is of little diagnostic value, but rhythm abnormalities would raise suspicion.
- Left ventricular and atrial enlargement pattern may be seen
- Arrhythmias: sinus tachycardia, ventricular and supraventricular premature complexes, occasionally atrial fibrillation
- Left anterior fascicular block is not uncommon

Radiography
- Cardiomegaly may or may not be evident
- Atrial enlargement is the usual cause of cardiomegaly and this can vary from mild to severe
- Biatrial enlargement may produce a 'valentine-shaped heart' on the DV view
- Signs of left-sided congestive failure:
  ○ Pulmonary vascular pattern (pulmonary venous enlargement)
  ○ Interstitial to alveolar pulmonary oedema
  ○ Pulmonary oedema can be of a widespread distribution
  ○ Patchy pleural effusion
- Signs of right-sided congestive failure:
  ○ Pleural effusion
  ○ Enlarged caudal vena cava
  ○ Hepatic enlargement, hepatic venous congestion

> **Note:** Pleural effusion can occur in cats with left-sided heart failure.

Echocardiography
Echocardiography is required to make a definitive diagnosis and assess severity, but changes vary considerably from the very mild and equivocal, to severe muscle-wall thickening, which is not necessarily symmetrical.
  ○ Left ventricular hypertrophy (concentric hypertrophy); wall thickness is not always uniform and it is not uncommon for the septum to be thicker than the free wall
  ○ End diastolic wall thickness >6 mm in cats (severe >8 mm)
- Need to rule out other potential causes of left ventricular hypertrophy:
  ○ HCM
  ○ Hyperthyroidism
  ○ Systemic hypertension
  ○ Aortic stenosis
  ○ Acromegaly

> **Note:** Wall thickness measurement is often easier and more reliable on a 2-D image than from an M-mode image.

- Papillary muscle hypertrophy
- Left ventricular chamber size is reduced
- Contractility is usually normal – fractional shortening percentage may be increased
- Left atrial dilation is often evident
- Mitral regurgitation is common
- Ball thrombi or spontaneous echocardiographic contrast (smoke) may be seen in the left atrium or auricle
- Doppler studies may demonstrate a decreased E to A ratio, or combined E and A waves
- Dynamic left ventricular outflow tract obstruction may be seen in some cats – *hypertrophic obstructive cardiomyopathy* (HOCM)
- Evidence of *myocardial infarction*

HYPERTROPHIC OBSTRUCTIVE CARDIOMYOPATHY (HOCM)

CLINICAL FINDINGS

Usually associated with a dynamic murmur – louder during periods of tachycardia, but becomes quiet when the heart rate reduces.

DIAGNOSIS

Echocardiography
- Ventricular septal hypertrophy
- During the course of systole the diameter of the *left ventricular outflow tract* (LVOT) decreases
- Velocity of blood ejected through LVOT then accelerates exponentially, which can be appreciated on spectral Doppler tracings
- At high velocities this causes the anterior cusp of the mitral valve to be drawn into the LVOT – *systolic anterior motion* (SAM) of the mitral valve
- This results in further narrowing of the LVOT and thus a further step up in ejection velocity (mid-systolic peak in velocity)
- The effect of this is greatest during period of tachycardia
- On M-mode tracings of the mitral valve (right short axis view) the septal leaflet can be seen to be displaced towards the septum during systole (when the valves should be closed)
- Colour Doppler studies (right long axis view) show two high-velocity turbulent jets arising from the same point, one associated with LVOT ejection and the other with mitral regurgitation because of SAM of the mitral valve

Dynamic testing of HOCM on echocardiography
- If HOCM is not evident at the time of echocardiography but is suspected, try increasing the cat's heart rate (make a noise)
- If the dynamic outflow tract obstruction is constantly present, try reducing the heart rate by patiently waiting for the cat to relax, or administer a beta blocker and repeat the scan after an appropriate time interval

THERAPY

There is such a spectrum of disease from mild to severe and from asymptomatic to symptomatic that there are no simple guidelines for treatment of HCM in cats.

Acute pulmonary oedema
- Cage rest and minimal manual restraint
- Furosemide at 1–2 mg/kg every 2–4 hours initially but reducing according to response:
  - Evidence of effective diuresis, i.e. urination
  - Improved respiration
  - Reduction in pulmonary crackles
- Nitroglycerine ointment – $1/4''$ applied to the skin, e.g. inside ear pinna
- Supplemental oxygen – without causing any stress or restraint

> **Note:** Diuresis in cats can easily result in dehydration, hypokalaemia and azotaemia.

Pleural effusion
- If causing respiratory distress requires thoracocentesis
- Furosemide and an ACE inhibitor are then required on an ongoing out-patient basis

Out-patient treatment

Cats are normally treated with as few medications as possible, most commonly just one or two drugs, typically an ACE inhibitor or beta blocker +/– furosemide.

Furosemide

- Oral dose is 1–2 mg/kg bid
- In cats with *Pulmonary oedema* – furosemide can often be weaned off (when also on ACE inhibitors)
- In cats with *Pleural effusion* – a low dose of furosemide is often required long term

ACE inhibitors (benazepril, ramipril, enalapril, imidapril)

- Useful in the management of congestive heart failure
- Thought to reduce myocardial fibrosis
- May be beneficial when there is myocardial ischaemia/infarction

β-blockers (propranolol, atenolol)

- Reduce the severity of dynamic obstruction in HOCM
- Help to control arrhythmias when present
- Beneficial if there is myocardial infarction

Calcium channel blockers (diltiazem)

- Reduce the severity of dynamic obstruction in HOCM
- Improve myocardial relaxation (lusitropy)
- Contraindicated when there is myocardial infarction

> **Note:** Use of glucocorticosteroids can precipitate or worsen congestive heart failure in cats.

PROGNOSIS

Mild cases of HCM may go undetected and cats can have a normal life expectancy. The outcome for mild to moderate cases of HCM is difficult to predict. Cats can remain asymptomatic for a long time (>3 years) or can present with peracute pulmonary oedema or thromboembolism.

Severe cases of HCM (LV wall thickness >8 mm and LA diameter >20 mm) often develop signs of congestive failure, thromboembolism or sudden death. For cats that present in congestive heart failure, the survival time is 3–18 months. Cats that present with thromboembolism have an approximate survival time of 2–6 months and recurrence is common.

RESTRICTIVE CARDIOMYOPATHY (RCM)

Restrictive cardiomyopathy probably accounts for up to one quarter of heart disease in adult cats and is characterised by decreased myocardial compliance (failure of relaxation). This restricts diastolic filling without left ventricular hypertrophy.

AETIOLOGY AND PATHOPHYSIOLOGY

- Unknown but may include: myocarditis, ischaemia/infarction
- Results in restricted diastolic filling and compliance
- Congestive heart failure arises as a result of elevated ventricular filling pressures

CLINICAL FINDINGS

- More common in middle-aged to older cats
- More likely to cause thromboembolism than HCM cases (see p. 114)

Common presentations
- Tachypnoea
- Dyspnoea due to peracute pulmonary oedema +/– pleural effusion
- Lethargy
- Inappetence
- Syncope – due to tachyarrhythmias
- Thromboembolism (see p. 114)

Clinical signs
- Heart sounds may be dulled by the presence of pleural effusion
- Distended jugular veins
- Arrhythmias – premature beats with pulse deficit
- Gallop sound
- Pulmonary crackles due to oedema
- Soft murmurs (grade 1–3) due to mitral regurgitation (best heard at the left apex or on the sternum)

DIAGNOSIS

Radiography
- Often moderate to marked atrial enlargement
- There may be generalised cardiomegaly
- Pulmonary oedema and/or pleural effusion

Electrocardiography
- Arrhythmias are common, typically supraventricular
- Left atrial and ventricular enlargement pattern

Echocardiography
- Ventricular septum and free-wall thickness may be within normal range
- Reduced ventricular wall motion (reduced fractional shortening)

- Left ventricular chamber dimensions are variable
- There may be an irregular-shaped ventricle and irregular echogenicities of the endocardium
- Severe atrial and auricular dilation
- Ball thrombi or 'smoke' may be evident
- Doppler evidence of diastolic dysfunction

THERAPY

Acute pulmonary oedema
- Cage rest and minimal manual restraint
- Furosemide at 1–2 mg/kg every 2–4 hours initially, but reducing according to response
  - Evidence of effective diuresis, i.e. urination
  - Improved respiration
  - Reduction in pulmonary crackles

> **Note:** Diuresis in cats can easily result in dehydration, hypokalaemia and azotaemia particularly cats with RCM.

- Nitroglycerine ointment – $1/4''$ applied to the skin, e.g. inside ear
- Supplemental oxygen – without causing any stress or restraint

Pleural effusion
- If causing respiratory distress, requires thoracocentesis
- Furosemide and an ACE inhibitor are then required on an ongoing out-patient basis

Out-patient treatment
Cats with RCM are normally given as few medications as possible, most commonly just one or two drugs, typically an ACE inhibitor or β-blocker +/– furosemide. Beta blockers or calcium channel blockers are generally not used in RCM, unless there are severe arrhythmias that require control.
- Furosemide
  - Oral dose is 1–2 mg/kg, reducing as congestive signs abate

○ Can be withdrawn (when also on ACE inhibitors) if *pulmonary oedema* only, but not if cat has *pleural effusion*
- ACE inhibitors (benazepril, ramipril, enalapril, imidapril)

PROGNOSIS

The prognosis is often poor, due to advanced nature of disease. Mean survival time is 4–5 months.

MYOCARDIAL INFARCTION IN FELINE CARDIOMYOPATHIES

This is probably an under-diagnosed complication
- Tends to affect left ventricular apex or free wall
- Echocardiography shows left ventricular dyskinesia and/or free-wall thinning; may result in reduced contractility
- Severe ventricular arrhythmias on ECG
- Grossly elevated serum troponin levels

UNCLASSIFIED CARDIOMYOPATHY IN CATS

In some cases it may not be possible to clearly categorise the type of cardiomyopathy (HCM, RCM, DCM) in cats. In such cases they are referred to as unclassified cardiomyopathy.

ATRIAL FIBROSIS/STANDSTILL

Atrial fibrosis/standstill is an uncommon condition in the Springer Spaniel, Old English Sheepdog and Cavalier King Charles Spaniel. It is very rare in cats. There are dilated, non-functional atria that are thin-walled and fibrotic. Disease is progressive with later ventricular involvement.

CLINICAL FEATURES

- Weakness, collapse or syncope
- Bilateral congestive heart failure may develop
- Murmurs of mitral and tricuspid valve regurgitation may be heard
- Bradycardia

DIAGNOSIS

ECG
- Atrial standstill
- Bradycardia

Echocardiography
- Dilated immobile atria
- No atrial contraction of AV valves evident on M-mode or on Doppler studies of ventricular inflow
- Progressive ventricular dilation develops

THERAPY

- Control signs of congestion
- Positive chronotropic drugs may be tried, e.g. theophylline or clenbuterol
- Pacemaker implantation is a debatable option, because of the progressive nature of the disease

PROGNOSIS

Prognosis is very poor, as disease is progressive.

FELINE ARTERIAL THROMBOEMBOLISM (FATE)

AETIOLOGY

Aortic thromboembolism is not an uncommon complication of cardiomyopathy in cats, usually in association with a dilated left atrium. A small percentage of cats presenting with thromboembolism do not show evidence of significant heart disease (<10%). Most emboli originate from a thrombus in the left atrium, with approximately 70% of emboli lodging in the distal aorta (*saddle thrombus*), but emboli may also lodge in a forelimb (brachial artery) and occasionally other sites, such as the kidneys, gut and brain.

The embolus obstructs blood flow through the affected artery/arteries, but, more important, results in constriction of collateral vessels due to release of vasoactive mediators (e.g. serotonin, thromboxane) producing an ischaemic neuromyopathy.

CLINICAL FINDINGS

Signs are acute with the following findings:
- Lameness with paresis or paralysis of the affected limb(s)
- Absence or very weak arterial pulses
- Nail beds or pads of the feet are pale +/− cyanotic and affected limbs are cold
- Affected limbs are painful, with the cat vocalising, unable to settle, rolling around and panting (or open-mouth breathing)
- Muscles of the affected limb are firm to palpate
- There are often also signs of systemic shock
  - Poor peripheral perfusion
  - Hypothermia (low rectal temperature is not specifically associated with embolism of the aortic bifurcation)

- Evidence of heart disease, with or without congestive heart failure, is often, but not always, present

DIAGNOSIS

- The history and clinical examination is usually sufficient to make a diagnosis
- Ultrasound examination of the distal aorta may demonstrate the thrombus and absence of flow – but this requires considerable operator skill
- Non-selective angiography may demonstrate the cessation or reduction in flow at the aorta

Clinical pathology
- Pre-renal azotaemia (urea elevated more than creatinine)
- Hyperglycaemia
- Elevated muscle enzymes (serum aspartate aminotransferase, creatine phosphokinase)

Common clinical findings
- Most commonly causes bilateral hind leg paresis (aortic/saddle thrombus)
- Sometimes results in paresis of a forelimb
- Absence of palpable pulse to affected limb (femoral or radial arteries)
- Pads of the foot or the nail beds become pale and/or cyanotic
- Limbs are palpably colder compared to non-affected limbs
- Limbs are often sore to palpate in the early stages

THERAPY

- Cage rest
- Analgesia: morphine (0.1 mg/kg), oxymorphone, fentanyl, butorphanol
- Treatment to prevent further thrombus formation in the early stages can be useful
  - Heparin (i/v or s/c) at 250 iu/kg every eight hours
- Management of congestive heart failure – this requires chest radiography to diagnose
  - Oxygen supplementation
  - Thoracocentesis if there is significant pleural effusion
  - Low-dose furosemide if there is pulmonary oedema
- Treatment of systemic signs of hypoperfusion (e.g. hypothermia)
  - Fluid therapy in dehydrated cats, if there are no signs of congestive heart failure
  - Nutritional support in anorexic cats
  - Avoid excessive external warming as this may result in peripheral vasodilation and shunting of blood and warmth away from vital organs
- Thrombolytic therapy can adversely affect outcome, because of associated limb ischaemia and resultant reperfusion injury, and is of doubtful or unproven benefit
  - Complications have included hyperkalaemia, haemorrhage and metabolic acidosis leading to death in many cases
  - If using thrombolytics, they should be used within 2–3 hours of the embolism occurring
    - Streptokinase: 90 000 iu over 30 minutes, then 45 000 iu/h for 3–6 h

- Treatments *not* recommended include:
  - Acepromazine, as it may exacerbate hypotension
  - Beta adrenoceptor blocking drugs, as these may enhance peripheral vasoconstriction

Long-term thrombus prevention

There is currently no evidence that thromboprophylaxis has long-term benefits

- Aspirin 5–30 mg twice a week is believed to be effective
- Warfarin: is difficult to use and has been associated with complications
- Low-molecular-weight heparins (need to be injected twice daily)
  - Enoxaparin 100 iu/kg s/c q12hr
  - Dalteparin 100–200 iu/kg s/c q12hr

Summary approach to managing feline aortic thromboembolism

- Analgesia, e.g. morphine
- Chest X-ray to screen for congestive heart failure
- Biochemistry and electrolytes
- Heparin 250 iu/kg every eight hours
- Oxygen supplementation
- I/v fluids if not in heart failure
- Nutritional support
- Cage rest in comfortable warm bedding without heat source

PROGNOSIS

Approximately one third of cats will die, one third will be euthanased and one third will survive to be discharged. Repeated events carry a very poor prognosis. Hypothermia and bradycardia on presentation are poor prognostic signs.

DISEASES OF THE CARDIORESPIRATORY SYSTEM

MYOCARDITIS

Myocarditis is defined as inflammation of the myocardium, and may be due to infectious or non-infectious causes. Definitive diagnosis of myocarditis is rarely made ante mortem. Serum troponin levels are usually markedly elevated, and often there are multiform ventricular premature complexes on ECG.

AETIOLOGY

INFECTIOUS CAUSES

Borrelia burgdorferi (borreliosis, Lyme carditis)
- Lyme disease is a tick-borne condition that causes:
  - Fever, lethargy, anorexia
  - Acute lameness, swollen painful joints
  - Skin lesions associated with the tick bite
  - Lymphadenopathy
  - Heart block and endocarditis
- Diagnosis is based on identifying a rising antibody titre and the disease can be effectively treated with tetracyclines or penicillins

Canine parvovirus
- Primarily a condition of young puppies (3–10 weeks old)
- Clinical features are not dissimilar to DCM
- Poor prognosis, usually fatal

Trypanosoma cruzi (Trypanosomiasis, Chagas' disease)
- A protozoal infection occuring in southeast United States, Central and South America and Africa
- Primarily a disease of dogs under two years old
- Acute and chronic forms seen
- Clinical signs are referrable to an infectious process and congestive heart failure
- Diagnosis requires demonstration of parasitaemia by culture, xenodiagnosis or serodiagnosis

NON-INFECTIOUS CAUSES

Ischaemic heart disease
- Coronary embolism
  - Infective endocarditis of the aortic valve
  - Septicaemia
  - Pulmonary neoplasia
  - Cardiomyopathy in cats
- Microscopic intramural myocardial infarction (MIMI)
  - Quite common in the dog
  - Clinical significance is questionable
  - May contribute to dysrhythmias
- Non-cardiac diseases
  - Gastric dilation-volvulus and acute necrotising pancreatitis etc.

Myocardial contusion
Physical injury to the heart may arise from trauma (traumatic myocarditis), e.g. road traffic accident, heat stroke or electric shock. Although other lesions may be more obvious, undetected cardiac trauma may result in death 12–24 hours after the trauma. ECG changes include ST segment elevation or depression and dysrhythmias, which may require treatment.

12 PERICARDIAL DISEASE AND CARDIAC NEOPLASIA

The pericardium envelops the heart and proximal portions of the great vessels. It consists of two membranes: a thin, *visceral pericardium* (epicardium), adherent to the myocardium, and a thicker, *parietal pericardium* (pericardial sac). The pericardial sac is normally a translucent, thin membranous tissue. Between these two membranes is the pericardial space, containing 1–15 ml of serous fluid.

Pericardial disease is uncommon, but probably the most common cause of isolated right-sided congestive heart failure in dogs. Pericardial disease is rare in the cat and is most likely to be secondary to cardiomyopathy or feline infectious peritonitis (FIP).

PERICARDIAL EFFUSION

AETIOLOGY (Table 12.1)

- Pericardial effusion is the most common consequence of diseases affecting the pericardium
- The majority of pericardial effusions are haemorrhagic (which is usually nonclotting)
- Can result in cardiac tamponade and clinical signs of forward heart failure and right-sided congestive failure
- The two most common causes of pericardial haemorrhage are:
  - Idiopathic pericarditis
  - Cardiac neoplasia
- Haemorrhage due to left atrial tear associated with gross left atrial dilation caused by mitral valve disease is infrequent; haemorrhage in this instance is rapid and leads either to death or an acute exacerbation of the heart failure
- A small to moderate volume of effusion can sometimes occur with congestive heart failure (in cats and dogs), but rarely causes tamponade
- A small effusion can occur secondary to hypoproteinaemia and usually does not cause cardiac tamponade
- Exudative (infectious) effusions are rare in small animals

PATHOPHYSIOLOGY

- Cardiac tamponade occurs when the intrapericardial pressure rises to a level greater than the right atrial and/or right ventricular diastolic pressures
- Increased pericardial pressure raises the intracardiac pressure which restricts right-sided diastolic filling
- In acute pericardial haemorrhage, 100 ml of effusion is sufficient to cause tamponade
- In chronic cases, effusions may gradually increase to amounts in excess of 1 litre; majority of cases present with 300–700 ml of fluid
- In recurrent cases the pericardium becomes fibrosed and restrictive (reduced compliance) so that a small effusion can lead to tamponade. This is referred to as *constrictive pericardial fibrosis*

TABLE 12.1   Aetiology of pericardial effusions

Type of Effusion	Aetiology
Transudate or Modified	• Hypoproteinaemia
Transudate	• Congestive heart failure • Peritoneopericardial diaphragmatic hernia

Haemorrhage	• Idiopathic pericarditis (benign pericardial effusion)
	• Neoplasia
	   ○ Haemangiosarcoma
	   ○ Heart base tumour
	• Left atrial rupture
	   ○ Secondary to mitral valve disease
	• Trauma
	   ○ External
	   ○ Iatrogenic

Exudate	• Infectious
	   ○ Penetrating FB
	   ○ Feline infectious peritonitis
	• Sterile
	   ○ Idiopathic
	   ○ Uraemic

Clinical features
- Similar, regardless of aetiology
- Can develop over a prolonged period
- Cardiac tamponade leads to:
  - Reduced cardiac output (forward failure signs)
  - More typically, reduced venous return and right-heart filling (right-sided congestive failure signs)

Clinical signs of pericardial effusion and cardiac tamponade
- Muffled heart sounds and reduced apex beat
- Weakness, lethargy
- Ascites and hepatomegaly
- Exercise intolerance
- Weak pulse +/− *pulsus paradoxus* (varies with respiration)
- Pallor
- Jugular distension
- Dyspnoea – usually related to pain
- Collapse – exacerbated by exertion
- Cough – in the initial period
- Vomiting and/or diarrhoea
- Polydipsia

CONDITIONS

Idiopathic pericarditis
- Non-clotting haemorrhagic pericardial effusion of unknown aetiology

- Synonymous terms are: idiopathic or benign pericardial haemorrhage
  - Medium to large-breed dogs
  - Middle-aged Golden Retrievers
  - Young (<3 years) St Bernards
  - More than 90% are male
  - The mean age is six years, with a range of 1–14 years
  - Up to one third develop constrictive pericardial fibrosis

Neoplastic disease

- The most common causes of pericardial effusion are:
  - Right atrial haemangiosarcoma
  - Aortic body tumour (chemodectoma)
  - Mesothelioma (uncommon)
- Occurs primarily in the older dog (average age is nine years, range 7–13 years)
- Occurs equally in males and females
- Haemangiosarcoma
  - Seen most commonly in the German Shepherd Dog
  - Usually located in the right atrium or its appendage and is highly malignant
- Heart-base tumours
  - Most common in Boxer dogs, but also seen in other brachycephalic breeds, e.g. Bulldog and Boston Terrier
- Mesothelioma
- Difficult to diagnose ante mortem
- May be a cause of persistent pleural effusions in some dogs following pericardiectomy

Differentiating between idiopathic pericarditis and cardiac neoplasia

- The effusion tends to develop more slowly in idiopathic pericarditis compared to neoplastic cases
- Ascites is more common in dogs with idiopathic pericarditis
- Collapse is more common in dogs with cardiac neoplasia
- Idiopathic pericarditis cases tend to have a larger volume

DIAGNOSIS

Clinical pathology

- Anaemia is found in one third of cases
- Low total proteins are seen in one quarter of cases, with globulins being low in nearly 50% of cases
- Pre-renal azotaemia may be present
- Liver enzymes may be raised

Pericardial fluid analysis

- Cytology of little diagnostic use to determine the aetiology, except if infection present
- Measurement of pH of little value

Electrocardiography

- Reduced R wave amplitude (less than 1 mV) in 50% of cases
- Electrical alternans in 30% of cases
- Ventricular premature complexes or ventricular tachycardia sometimes present
- A rising ST segment, or elevated ST segment is occasionally present

Radiography

- Cardiac silhouette is usually enlarged and globular in shape in both the lateral and DV views, with a sharp outline; the presence of pleural effusion can mask this
- There is often evidence of right-sided congestive heart failure
  - Widening of the caudal vena cava
  - Hepatomegaly and/or ascites
  - Pleural effusion
- Large heart base tumours might be detected with mediastinal widening and displacement of the trachea or cranial-lobe bronchi
- Definitive diagnosis can be difficult with radiography alone

Echocardiography

- This is the most effective diagnostic procedure
- Fluid is visualised between the heart and pericardium

- Cardiac tamponade is evident as intermittent collapse of the right atrial and/or right ventricular walls
- Tumours (masses) are usually easier to identify prior to pericardiocentesis, but cannot be discounted if not seen
- Right atrial haemangiosarcoma is seen on the right parasternal short axis or the left caudal parasternal four chamber views
- An aortic body tumour may been seen adjacent to, or surrounding, the ascending aorta

THERAPY

- Cardiac tamponade is treated by pericardiocentesis (see below). The volume of effusion in dogs with idiopathic pericarditis is approximately 400–900 ml and in dogs with tumours is 250–600 ml
- Following pericardiocentesis, removing at least one quarter of the effusion, most dogs will show a good clinical improvement over the subsequent 3–5 days
- Any ascites resolves over a few days following pericardiocentesis, without the need for diuresis, because of the improvement in cardiac output
- Vasodilators or diuretics are contraindicated as they can cause hypotension
- A subtotal pericardiectomy is indicated for dogs with recurrent pericardial effusions and/or constrictive pericardial fibrosis
- Pericardial effusions that are secondary to other diseases (e.g. cardiomyopathy, hypoproteinaemia) usually respond to treatment of the primary cause, while surgical excision of tumours is either unnecessary or unsuccessful

> **Note:** Dogs in cardiogenic shock due to cardiac tamponade require rapid i/v fluids.

TECHNIQUE FOR PERICARDIOCENTESIS

- The technique described here uses a set designed for this purpose, the Martin Pericardiocentesis Catheter Set (Global Veterinary Products). This catheter is less suitable for small effusions, such as occur with constrictive pericardial fibrosis
- Alternatively, one can use large i/v catheters or over-the-needle catheters, jugular catheter sets

Equipment
- Local anaesthesia (2% lignocaine)
- No. 11 scalpel blade for stab skin incision
- 20 ml and 50 ml syringes
- 3-way tap and collecting container
- Sterile window drape
- ECG monitor
- Martin Pericardiocentesis Catheter Set

Preparation of dog
- Obtain peripheral blood and check PCV
- Analgesia and sedation (0.01–0.02 mg/kg ACP + 0.5 mg/kg morphine i/m)
- Place the dog in left lateral recumbency and attach the ECG monitor
- Clip and surgically prepare the area of the right cardiac apex, i.e. 5th–6th intercostal spaces at the level of the costochondral junctions (double check position by ultrasound examination if required)
- Infiltrate local anaesthesia into the site of puncture and deep to the pleura

Procedure
- Make a stab incision through the skin and partially through the intercostal muscle at the site of local anaesthesia
- Attach a 20 ml syringe to the needle, insert the needle through the stab incision and into the pleural cavity
- Redirect the needle so that it is perpendicular to the pericardium – this usually means directing towards the heart

- Maintaining a small vacuum on the 20 ml syringe, advance the needle until pericardial effusion (usually a bloody effusion) is withdrawn. *If the needle touches the heart it may result in ectopics or a change in the ST segment*
- Holding the needle in this position, remove the syringe and insert the guide wire (soft-end) through the needle and into the pericardium
- Remove the needle, leaving the guide wire positioned in the pericardium
- Thread the catheter over the guide wire, through the skin and intercostal space and into the pericardium, continually rotating it around the guide wire
- Remove the guide wire, leaving the catheter in the pericardium
- Attach a 50 ml syringe and 3-way tap to the catheter and withdraw the pericardial effusion. If this is a bloody effusion, and you are not certain it is pericardial (versus cardiac blood), check the PCV and clotting time of the effusion. The PCV is usually very different and the pericardial effusion does not clot

- Continue to withdraw all the pericardial effusion gently and then remove the catheter, suturing the skin incision

PROGNOSIS

- Neoplasia cases rarely survive more than two months, although, with an aortic body tumour, pericardiectomy is an option and can improve survival (median of 24 months)
- 50% of dogs with idiopathic pericarditis will have a recurrence, typically within months, but up to four years after pericardiocentesis. Many can have a third recurrence, necessitating a subtotal pericardiectomy. Pericardiectomy results in a long-term survival rate of about 80%, with such dogs surviving twice as long as those not having a pericardiectomy. The perioperative death rate is approximately 10%
- Idiopathic persistent pleural effusion can develop post-operatively in up to 10% of dogs, and usually leads to euthanasia

INFECTIOUS PERICARDITIS

- Primarily a problem of dogs, but very rare
- Usually occurs following a penetrating foreign body injury leading to a bacterial pericarditis
- Diagnosis is by cytological examination of the effusion (with cell count), and irregular echogenicities on echocardiography

- Treatment is by pericardiocentesis and prolonged high-dose antibiotic therapy
- Surgical exploration, with excision of the pericardium, may be a consideration in some cases
- Prognosis is poor

CONGENITAL DISORDERS OF THE PERICARDIUM

PERITONEOPERICARDIAL DIAPHRAGMATIC HERNIA

- In this defect there is a persistent communication between the pericardial and peritoneal cavities, which permits

abdominal organs to enter the pericardial sac
- The extent of herniation is variable and clinical signs may occur within weeks of birth or after several years
- Signs may never appear

- The Weimaraner appears to be predisposed and it is not uncommon in the cat
- The clinical signs may be gastrointestinal (vomiting, diarrhoea, anorexia, weight loss) and/or respiratory (dyspnoea, cough)
- Diagnosis is made by radiography and ultrasound
- Treatment is by surgical correction of the hernia and, in uncomplicated cases, carries a good prognosis
- Occasionally the liver may be adhesed to the pericardium and the prognosis in such cases is guarded

PERICARDIAL CYSTS

- These are usually found at the apex of the parietal pericardium, usually lying within the pericardial space
- The clinical signs may be similar to pericardial effusion and treatment is by surgical excision, which carries a good prognosis

13 CONGENITAL HEART DISEASE

- The prevalence of congenital heart disease in dogs and cats is estimated to be <1% of the population.
- Innocent systolic murmurs are common in very young dogs and cats, usually disappear by 4–6 months of age and need to be considered in any list of differential diagnoses for this age group.

TABLE 13.1 Common congenital defects in dogs and cats

Dogs	Cats
Patent ductus arteriosus (PDA)	Ventricular septal defect
Aortic stenosis	Atrioventricular valve dysplasia
Pulmonic stenosis	

PATENT DUCTUS ARTERIOSUS (PDA)

- One of the three most common congenital defects in dogs; uncommon in cats
- Females are affected twice as often as males
- The 50% survival rate is less than one year
- The majority of dogs progress into left-sided congestive failure
- Reverse shunting is rare. It will rarely occur after six months of age

BREEDS OF DOG WITH A HIGH PREVALENCE OF PDA

- German Shepherd Dog
- Border Collie
- Cavalier King Charles Spaniel
- Poodle
- Shetland Sheepdog
- Cocker Spaniel
- Pomeranian
- Irish Setter

AETIOLOGY

- Failure of the ductus arteriosus to close fully at or shortly after birth
- Believed to be an inherited defect (polygenic transmission)

PATHOPHYSIOLOGY

- Shunting of blood from the higher pressure aorta to the pulmonary artery.
- Increased volume of blood passing through the lungs and returning to the left heart.
- Left atrial (and ventricular) dilation, increased LA pressure, increased PV pressure and, ultimately, pulmonary congestion (left-sided congestive heart failure).
- Should pulmonary hypertension occur (rare) and the pulmonary artery pressure

exceed that of the aorta, the murmur can disappear (reverse shunting PDA). Blood then bypasses the lungs and the patient presents with caudal (differential) cyanosis and, in time, a compensatory polycythaemia.

CLINICAL FEATURES

There is a pathognomonic continuous murmur, which increases in intensity during systole.

- Usually grade 5 with a palpable precordial thrill
- The diastolic component of the murmur can be easily missed if the stethoscope is not placed near to the PDA (high and well forward on the left thorax)
- The femoral pulse is often hyperkinetic (hyperdynamic)
- Most young dogs will present as asymptomatic; many are thin or smaller than siblings
- Signs of forward and/or left-sided congestive heart failure (see Chapter 6)

DIAGNOSIS

Differentials

Differentials for a 'continuous' murmur are:

- Aberrant bronchoesophageal artery
- Aorticopulmonary window
- Aortic stenosis with aortic regurgitation
- Ventricular septal defect with aortic regurgitation
- Pulmonic stenosis with pulmonic regurgitation

ECG

- Not specific, although there are often very tall QRS complexes
- Supraventricular arrhythmias such as atrial fibrillation may occur

Radiography

- Pulmonary over-circulation (dilated pulmonary arteries and veins)
- Left atrial dilation is common
- Sometimes (25% of cases) bulging of the aorta and pulmonary arteries and left atrial dilation, resulting in three bulges in the cardiac silhouette on the DV view, at the 1, 2 and 3 o'clock positions respectively
- Signs of left CHF develop in most cases if left untreated

Angiography

- Routinely performed prior to interventional closure
- Reveals the location, size and shape (type) of ductus

Echocardiography

- LA dilation is fairly common
- Mitral regurgitation is often present secondary to annular dilation
- LV dilation is often present with hyperdynamic contractility
- The ductus is difficult to visualise, but can often be seen on the left cranial short axis view
- Doppler echocardiography will reveal the continuous flow from the ductus within the pulmonary artery, with the maximal systolic velocity approaching 5 m/s (if there is no pulmonary hypertension)

THERAPY

- Closure/ligation of the ductus is the treatment of choice
  - Traditional surgery via a lateral thoracotomy and direct duct ligation
  - Interventional transcatheter techniques (keyhole surgery), occluding the duct with either coils or an Amplatzer duct occluder (Figure 13.1)

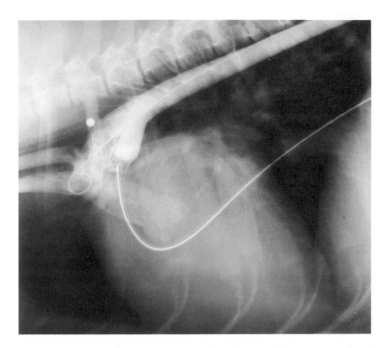

FIGURE 13.1 Angiogram demonstrating good occlusion and positioning of an Amplatzer Duct Occluder (ADO) in a patent ductus arteriosus from an 11 month old German Shephard dog. Note the contrast, injected via the pigtail catheter, filling the aorta and part of the duct, but absence of contrast passing through the duct into the pulmonary artery. The delivery wire is still attached to the ADO. The ball bearing in the tip of the oesophageal stethoscope acts as a scale for measurement purposes.

- Treatment of signs of congestive failure (if present) prior to anaesthesia (see Chapter 6, p. 68)
- Closure/ligation is contraindicated when the PDA is reverse shunting (right-to-left) or when there is severe left ventricular myocardial failure

PROGNOSIS

- Excellent with successful closure/ligation, although there is a documented 5–8% mortality rate for the traditional surgical method
- The prognosis without surgery is considered very poor in the majority of cases

REVERSE SHUNTING DEFECTS AND POLYCYTHAEMIA

- Reverse shunting occurs with tetralogy of Fallot and, uncommonly, with a PDA or VSD in which pulmonary hypertension develops (Eisenmenger's physiology)
- This leads to a systemic hypoxia/cyanosis which triggers erythropoesis and ultimately a polycythaemia
- The polycythaemia can be managed

by regular phlebotomy (although this seems to exacerbate the erythropoesis) or by the use of hydroxycarbamide

Use of hydroxycarbamide to control polycythaemia

- Hydroxycarbamide (hydroxyurea) comes as 500 mg tablets (Hydrea, Squibb)
- Dose for polycythaemia is approximately 50 mg/kg twice a week to start
- Monitor haematology, initially weekly
- The dose, or its frequency, is halved when the desired PCV is reached, and thereafter adjusted according to the rise and fall of the PCV (target <60–65%)

- Side effects include myelosuppression (neutropaenia, thrombocytopaenia) – hence the full haematology; if this occurs, the drug should be stopped until there is an improvement, then re-started
- Other side effects include anorexia or vomiting and, rarely, toenail sloughing or loss of hair on the flanks

Caution: This is a cytotoxic drug and should be handled with great care. Gloves should be worn and pregnant women should not handle it. All contaminated material should be disposed of as clinical waste.

AORTIC STENOSIS

Aortic stenosis is one of the three most common defects in dogs. It is uncommon in cats.

BREEDS OF DOG WITH A HIGH PREVALENCE OF AORTIC STENOSIS

- Boxer
- Golden Retriever
- Newfoundland
- German Shepherd Dog
- Rottweiller
- English Bull Terrier
- Samoyed

AETIOLOGY

- Inherited in Newfoundlands and likely to be inherited in other breeds
- The lesion occurs in three forms:
  - Supravalvular (rare)
  - Valvular (uncommon)
  - Subvalvular fibrous ring (subaortic stenosis – the most common form)

PATHOPHYSIOLOGY

- Restricts outflow and thus cardiac output, particular during periods of high demand such as exercise
- The left ventricular myocardium hypertrophies in proportion to the severity of the stenosis
- Excessive hypertrophy leads to ischaemia of the endomyocardial zone, resulting in ectopic foci that generate tachyarrhythmias
- Tachyarrhythmias may result in syncope or sudden death
- Vasovagal syncope may be more common in Boxers with aortic stenosis through pressure activation of ventricular mechanoreceptors (on exertion/excitement) and inappropriate vasodilation and bradycardia
- The mitral valve rarely becomes incompetent, despite the elevated left ventricular pressures and left-sided congestive heart failure is uncommon

TABLE 13.2 Classification of the severity of aortic stenosis

Severity	Trans-stenotic Pressure Gradient	Prognosis
Mild	<50 mmHg	Likely to remain asymptomatic and live a full and normal life
Moderate	50–100 mmHg	May develop symptoms in the latter half of life
Severe	>100 mmHg	Likely to become symptomatic in the first half of life and at high risk from sudden death

CLINICAL FEATURES

- Can vary from asymptomatic to exercise intolerance, syncope and sudden death
- The majority of cases are asymptomatic and a murmur is the only finding
- Murmur
  - Harsh systolic murmur, point of maximum intensity over the left heart base;
  - May radiate up the carotids and to the right side of the thorax
  - The grade of murmur is proportional to the severity of the stenosis
  - The lesion of subaortic stenosis may progress in severity within the first 6–12 months of life and the murmur may become louder in this time

DIAGNOSIS

ECG

If there is marked left ventricular hypertrophy, there may be tall and prolonged QRS complexes with a left axis deviation and/or ventricular arrhythmias (e.g. ventricular premature complexes)

Radiography

- Usually no enlargement of the cardiac silhouette on radiographs
- A post-stenotic bulge in the aorta may be evident on the DV view

Echocardiography

- A subaortic fibrous lesion may be evident
- In severe cases, there is left ventricular hypertrophy
- A post-stenotic bulge is sometimes seen
- Doppler studies are the definitive means of diagnosis and assessment of severity
  - Ideally performed via the subcostal view for best alignment to flow
  - Demonstrates an increase in velocity through the stenosis, from which the pressure gradient is estimated (using the Bernoulli equation) (Table 13.2)

THERAPY

Treatment is usually required only in moderately or severely affected cases and those showing clinical signs.

Medical treatment

- β-blockers, e.g. propranolol or atenolol, starting at low doses, may help to reduce the outflow obstruction
- For control of ventricular arrhythmias, β-blockers or mexiletine

Balloon catheter dilation

Can produce a reduction in pressure gradient, but long-term benefit is not well documented.

DISEASES OF THE CARDIORESPIRATORY SYSTEM

Surgical valve replacement

Resection of the subaortic fibrous ring and aortic valve replacement is possible, however there are few published data on success rates.

PROGNOSIS

- The majority of dogs have mild aortic stenosis and will live a full and normal life
- In more severe cases, clinical signs and prognosis are dictated by the severity (Table 13.2)

PULMONIC STENOSIS

Pulmonic stenosis is one of the three most common congenital defects in dogs. It is uncommon in cats.

BREEDS OF DOG WITH A HIGH PREVALENCE OF PULMONIC STENOSIS

- Labrador
- Cocker Spaniel
- English Bulldog
- Yorkshire Terrier
- Boxer
- Shih Tzu
- Cavalier King Charles Spaniel
- Mastiff
- Samoyed
- Miniature Schnauzer
- West Highland White Terrier
- Chow Chow
- Beagle

AETIOLOGY

- Inherited in the Beagle (polygenic trait) and likely to be hereditary in other breeds
- Supravalvular (rare), valvular (the most common form) and subvalvular forms
- The pathology of valvular stenosis is a mix of:
  - Commissural fusion of the cusps
  - Valve dysplasia
  - Annular hypoplasia

- In some dogs, e.g. English Bulldogs, with a subvalvular stenosis there is an anomalous left main coronary artery which encircles the outflow tract within the stenosis, and this prevents balloon valvuloplasty being undertaken

PATHOPHYSIOLOGY

- Restricts right ventricular outflow and so affects cardiac output, particularly on exertion
- Right ventricular hypertrophy
- 10–20% of dogs may have concurrent tricuspid dysplasia, leading to tricuspid valve regurgitation, right atrial dilation and ultimately right-sided congestive heart failure

CLINICAL FEATURES

- Asymptomatic through to exercise intolerance and syncope
- A systolic murmur may be the only finding, usually heard maximally over the left heart base
- If there is concurrent tricuspid valve regurgitation then right-sided congestive heart failure is also likely, in which case there will also be a systolic murmur on the right side of the thorax due to tricuspid regurgitation

SECTION 3

TABLE 13.3 Classification of the severity of pulmonic stenosis

Severity	Trans-stenotic Pressure Gradient	Prognosis
Mild	<40 mmHg	Likely to remain asymptomatic and live a full and normal life
Moderate	40–80 mmHg	Clinical signs are unlikely to occur, but may do so in the latter half of life
Severe	>80 mmHg	Likely to become symptomatic in the first half of life and at high risk from sudden death. Balloon valvuloplasty is indicated

DIAGNOSIS

ECG

- With marked right ventricular hypertrophy there is usually a right ventricular enlargement pattern with a right axis deviation
- Ventricular tachyarrhythmias (ventricular premature complexes) may be present in more severely affected cases
- Tall P wave if there is tricuspid valve incompetence

Radiography

- Right ventricular enlargement may be seen
- Post-stenotic bulging in the pulmonary artery may be evident
- Right atrial enlargement may be present in cases with tricuspid regurgitation

Angiography

- Routinely performed prior to balloon valvuloplasty
- Reveals the location and severity of the stenosis

Echocardiography

- Right ventricular hypertrophy in severe cases
- Flattening of the interventricular septum

- Abnormal pulmonary valves often evident, with a post-stenotic bulge in the pulmonary artery trunk
- Right atrial enlargement if there is tricuspid valve regurgitation
- Doppler studies for definitive diagnosis and assessment of severity
  - Increase in velocity through the stenosis, from which the pressure gradient is estimated (Table 13.3)
  - Pulmonic valve incompetence is commonly present
  - Identification of dynamic outflow tract obstruction
  - Identification of tricuspid valve regurgitation
  - A patent *foramen ovale* is not an uncommon concurrent finding; echocontrast study may be useful to screen for right-to-left shunting

Note: Right ventricular systolic pressure should work out to be the same when estimated from either the tricuspid regurgitation or the pulmonic stenosis

THERAPY

Treatment is usually required only in moderately or severely affected cases and those showing clinical signs.

Medical treatment

- Beta-adrenoreceptor blockers
  - When there is dynamic outflow tract obstruction
  - Beneficial in reducing arrhythmias prior to balloon valvuloplasty
- ACE inhibitor and furosemide if there is right-sided congestive heart failure

Balloon valvuloplasty

- Balloon valvuloplasty reduces the severity of the stenosis – it does not produce a 'cure'
- Balloon valvuloplasty has now mostly superseded surgical treatment
- Successful valvuloplasty results in a reduction in pressure gradient of >50% and provides a good, long-term clinical outcome (improvement in exercise tolerance and in life expectancy) in 85% of cases

- The operative mortality rate is approximately 5–7%
- Balloon valvuloplasty is less successful in cases of annular hypoplasia

Indications

- Presence of clinical signs (regardless of pressure gradient)
- Doppler derived trans-stenotic pressure gradient >80 mmHg
- Severe right ventricular hypertrophy with dynamic outflow tract obstruction

PROGNOSIS

- A prognosis can be offered based upon severity (Table 13.3)
- The presence of concurrent tricuspid dysplasia and right-sided congestive failure warrants a more guarded prognosis

VENTRICULAR SEPTAL DEFECT (VSD)

Ventricular septal defect (VSD) is one of the more common defects in cats, but is uncommon in dogs. In cats it is often associated with defects of the atrial septum or atrioventricular valves. There is no strong breed prevalance, but some breeds in which it has been reported are:

- Border Terrier
- Border Collie
- English Bulldog
- Keeshond
- Springer Spaniel
- West Highland White Terrier

PATHOPHYSIOLOGY

- A VSD results in shunting of blood from the left to right ventricles
- Volume overload of the pulmonary circulation and thus the left heart, that might result in left-sided congestive heart failure
- Occasionally, with large VSDs, pulmonary hypertension may develop (*Eisenmenger's syndrome*) causing a pressure overload of the right ventricle, and flow may become bidirectional or completely reversed

AETIOLOGY

- The majority of VSDs are high in the septum, i.e. subaortic or perimembranous
- Muscular VSDs, located lower in the septum, are rare in small animals

CLINICAL FEATURES

- Loud, harsh, systolic murmur heard maximally over the right thorax, typically on the cranial sternal border
- Usually asymptomatic, unless left-sided congestive heart failure develops (rare)

SECTION 3

DIAGNOSIS

Radiography
Radiographic findings are variable, due to the variation in severity of VSDs.
- Over-circulation of the pulmonary vessels may be evident
- Left atrial (and left ventricular) enlargement appear to be quite common
- Enlargement of the pulmonary artery may be seen on the DV view
- If pulmonary hypertension develops (rare) then right heart enlargement will be evident

Echocardiography
- Moderate to large VSDs are often seen on 2-D echocardiography but small VSDs (<2 mm) can be difficult to visualise
- There is often dilation (volume loading) of the left atrium and ventricle
- Doppler used to identify the blood flow through the VSD and measure the velocities across it (maximal systolic velocity approaching 5 m/s)

Note: The normal membranous portion of the high ventricular septum can give the false positive diagnosis of a VSD due to 'echo-drop out' by the thin membrane.

THERAPY
- Ideally, treatment involves open heart surgery and patch closure of the VSDs
- Interventional closure using Amplatzer devices is now being used in children and this may become possible for dogs with advances in this specialist field
- Palliative surgery can be performed by pulmonary artery banding to restrict the over-circulation of the lungs
- Congestive heart failure is managed medically (see Chapter 6)

PROGNOSIS
- A small VSD (which produces a high velocity jet and consequently a loud murmur) can be well tolerated and associated with a normal life
- Some small VSDs (diameter <2 mm) in young animals may close with growth to adulthood
- If the defect is <40% the diameter of the aorta, the prognosis is likely to be good
- Large defects are associated with volume over-loading of the left heart and left-sided congestive failure.

ATRIOVENTRICULAR (MITRAL AND TRICUSPID) VALVE DYSPLASIA

AETIOLOGY

- Congenital abnormalities of the mitral and tricuspid valves are seen in both the dog and cat
- Likely to have a genetic basis
- Larger breed dogs appear to be more commonly affected
  - Great Dane
  - German Shepherd Dog
  - Labrador Retriever
  - Old English Sheepdog
  - English Bull Terrier (sometimes also with mitral stenosis)
- In the Labrador, tricuspid valve dysplasia is often also associated with a re-entrant supraventricular tachycardia (SVT), which can result in episodic weakness

PATHOPHYSIOLOGY

The abnormal valves result in regurgitation, producing marked atrial dilation leading to atrial arrhythmias and also ventricular dilation. They can eventually result in left- or right-sided congestive heart failure.

CLINICAL FEATURES

- Systolic murmur heard over the affected valve (left apex for the mitral valve and right mid-heart area for the tricuspid valve)
- Progression to congestive heart failure is common, with the typically associated clinical signs

DIAGNOSIS

ECG
- Atrial and/or ventricular enlargement patterns may be seen
- Atrial premature complexes or tachycardia, and atrial fibrillation
- Some Labradors may also have a concurrent SVT, thought to be associated with a macrore-entry bypass tract

Radiography
Radiographic findings are atrial and/or ventricular enlargement and the associated findings of left- and/or right-sided congestive heart failure.

Echocardiography
- Abnormally-shaped valve cusps, *chordae tendineae* or papillary muscles on 2-D echocardiography (although such abnormalities can be difficult to appreciate on echocardiography)
- Regurgitant flow identified on Doppler

THERAPY

- Treatment is aimed at the signs of congestive failure (see Chapter 6) and is similar to treatment for chronic valvular disease seen in adult dogs
- Surgical correction or valve replacement might become an option in the future

PROGNOSIS

- The majority of dogs with mitral dysplasia develop arrhythmias and/or heart failure within the first year of life, but this will depend on the severity of the lesion
- In contrast, tricuspid dysplasia is better tolerated and dogs may live for many years, unless complicated by a concurrent re-entrant SVT
- Cats may live almost normal lives and survive for several years, probably partly due to their sedentary life style

TETRALOGY OF FALLOT

This is a rare congenital abnormality that results in shunting of blood from right to left and consequently hypoxaemia, exercise intolerance and cyanosis. It consists of:

(1) Subaortic VSD (usually large)

(2) Right ventricular outflow obstruction (in some severe forms there is pulmonary artery hypoplasia or atresia)

(3) Dextropositioned (or over-riding) aorta

(4) Secondary right ventricular hypertrophy

PATHOPHYSIOLOGY

- Right-to-left blood flow through the VSD results in desaturated blood being shunted into the aorta, leading to systemic hypoxaemia, cyanosis and compensatory polycythaemia
- Animals become incapacitated by hypoxia as opposed to congestive heart failure

CLINICAL FEATURES

- Animals are usually stunted in growth
- Exercise intolerance, syncope, tachypnoea and cyanosis
- Murmur of pulmonic stenosis
- The packed cell volume is usually elevated and may be in excess of 75%

DIAGNOSIS

Radiography
- Rounding of the right ventricular border
- Pulmonary vessels are under-perfused
- A pulmonic bulge may be evident on a lateral view

Angiography
Non-selective – shows shunting of blood from the right ventricle into the aorta.

Echocardiography
- Right ventricular hypertrophy
- Small left heart
- Large subaortic VSD
- Right ventricular outflow obstruction
- Pulmonic stenosis and reverse shunting VSD
- Echo-contrast studies (see Chapter 4) are useful to confirm the right-to-left shunt

THERAPY

- Exercise restriction is important
- Surgical palliation can be provided by creating a systemic-to-pulmonary shunt, to increase pulmonary perfusion (anastomosing a subclavian artery to a pulmonary artery)
- β-blockers – may minimise the right ventricular hypertrophy
- Phlebotomy and fluid replacement is necessary to control a severe compensatory polycythaemia – PCV is usually maintained at less than 65% (see Reverse shunting defects and polycythaemia above)

PROGNOSIS

- The prognosis is very poor for these cases; sudden death is common
- Surgical palliation, if successful, may provide relief of clinical signs for four years or longer

ATRIAL SEPTAL DEFECT

Atrial septal defect (ASD) is less commonly recognised in small animals, probably because it rarely produces clinical signs. It is more common in the cat than the dog.

The aetiology is unknown and ASD is more commonly recognised as a complication of other congenital heart defects. Treatment is rarely required.

14 PARASITIC DISEASE

LUNGWORM

The lungworm parasites are from the metastrongylid group. Foxes often act as a reservoir of infection for canines. The lung parasites of importance in the dog are: *Angiostrongylus vasorum, Crenosoma vulpis, Oslerus (Filaroides) osleri*. The main lung parasite of importance in the cat is *Aelurostrongylus abstrusus*. Other parasites include *Capillaria aerophilia* and *Paragonimus kellicotti*, but they are not present in the British Isles. *Filaroides hirthi* can cause pneumonitis.

ANGIOSTRONGYLUS VASORUM

Angiostrongylus vasorum parasitises the pulmonary artery and its branches, but is also found in the right ventricle. It causes significant and frequent disease in south-west France, but has also been recorded in Uganda, Spain, Denmark, Turkey, Brazil, Panama State, Ireland, the UK and occasionally the USA.

AETIOPATHOGENESIS

- Adult worms parasitise the pulmonary artery and right ventricle and lay eggs in the pulmonary parenchyma
- First-stage larvae (L1) enter the airways and are coughed up, swallowed and passed in the faeces
- Snails or slugs act as intermediate hosts
- Infection is by eating infected snails or slugs
- The pre-patent period is approximately 50–60 days.

CLINICAL FEATURES

- Dogs tend to be between four months and four and half years of age and often reared outdoors in runs
- Clinical signs are variable, partly depending upon the level of infection, and many cases are subclinical
- Coughing is the most common clinical presentation
- Additional clinical signs include:
  ○ Weakness
  ○ Subcutaneous swelling (haematoma)
  ○ Lameness
  ○ Anaemia
  ○ Pulmonary crepitation
  ○ Right-sided heart failure
  ○ Collapse
  ○ Dyspnoea and respiratory distress
  ○ Emaciation
  ○ Stunting
  ○ Poor performance
- Lumbar pain, hind leg paresis and intracranial haemorrhage have been reported, with associated neurological signs

Table 14.1 Treatment of lungworm infection with fenbendazole

Level of Infection	Dose
Mild	100 mg/kg daily for 5–7 days
Moderate	50 mg/kg daily for 7–10 days
Severe	20 mg/kg daily for 10–14 days

DIAGNOSIS

Clinical pathology
- Circulatory and pulmonary eosinophilia
- Abnormal coagulation profiles and thrombocytopaenia not uncommon
- Anaemia in some cases
- Hypercalcaemia occasionally
- L1 may be found in faeces or bronchoalveolar lavage (BAL) samples, but their absence does not preclude infection

Radiography
- A mixed pattern (predominantly bronchointerstitial) with patchy alveolar areas, particularly in the dorsocaudal lung field
- Right heart enlargement may also be noted

THERAPY

- Fenbendazole is currently the drug of choice (Table 14.1)
- If there is a deterioration in signs after 2–3 doses of fenbendazole, postpone further medication, give daily injections of dexamethasone until there is a remission and then restart the fenbendazole
- Other benzimadazole anthelmintics and avermectins may also be effective

PROGNOSIS

The prognosis for subclinical and mildly affected cases is good, with a good response to treatment. More severely affected cases may develop respiratory problems. Pulmonary thromboembolism may lead to death.

CRENOSOMA VULPIS

AETIOLOGY

- Parasitises the airways predominantly
- Snails or slugs act as intermediate hosts
- Pathology is similar to angiostrongylosis

CLINICAL FEATURES

- Dogs of any age can be affected
- Variable clinical signs and many cases are subclinical

- Coughing is the most common clinical presentation
- Dyspnoea may occur

DIAGNOSIS

Clinical pathology
- Circulatory and pulmonary eosinophilia are common
- L1 may be found in the faeces or bronchial washings

- L1 or adults can also be found in bronchial washings

Radiography

Mixed pattern, with a patchy alveolar density and a diffuse interstitial pattern. Pulmonary congestion and right heart enlargement may also be noted.

TREATMENT

As for angiostrongylosis.

PROGNOSIS

The prognosis for subclinical and mildly affected cases is good, with a good response to treatment. More severely affected cases may develop respiratory problems.

OSLERUS (FILAROIDES) OSLERI

AETIOPATHOGENESIS

- Primarily affects dogs under two years of age
- Dam to offspring transmission through oral and faecal contamination
- Usually infected within the first eight weeks of life

CLINICAL FEATURES

- Coughing
- In severe cases *Oslerus osleri* nodules may cause airway obstruction and respiratory distress
- Anorexia, debility and cachexia can occur, but rarely.

DIAGNOSIS

Clinical pathology
- Circulating eosinophilia possible
- Airway eosinophilia very likely finding
- Demonstration of larvae in faecal samples (often negative) or larvae or embryonated eggs in airway washes

Radiography
Often of little value in *Oslerus osleri* infection, with no identifiable changes seen.

Bronchoscopy
Visualisation of nodules at the carina.

TREATMENT

- As for angiostrongylosis
- Scraping or removal of nodules may be necessary when they are causing airway obstruction

AELUROSTRONGYLUS ABSTRUSUS

- Relatively rare, may be more common in cats eating prey (rodents, birds)
- Majority of infected individuals probably remain asymptomatic
- Indirect life cycle – pass through intermediate molluscan and paratenic (birds and small mammals palatable to the cat) hosts
- Clinical signs often self limiting in 6–9 months, but can be similar to feline asthma
- Treatment as angiostrongylosis

HEARTWORM

DIROFILARIASIS

Dirofilaria immitis infection is the most commonly recognised heartworm infection of dogs. It is enzootic in much of the tropical and sub-tropical areas of the world, including Australia, Japan and along the Atlantic coastline and Mississippi river in the USA. However, the parasite is becoming more adaptable and infection is spreading to more temperate climates. A low incidence of infection can be found in many areas of the USA and even Canada.

AETIOLOGY

- Transmission by third-stage larvae (L3) is by blood-sucking mosquitoes, which act as both intermediate host and vector
- The adult worms eventually end up in the pulmonary artery and also the right heart
- The adult worms are large (females 23–31 cm and males 15–19 cm in length)
- Pre-patent period takes up to 190 days
- Microfilariae (L1) undergo two moults in the mosquito and then migrate to the mouth parts as L3 (10–14 days)

PATHOLOGY AND PATHOPHYSIOLOGY

- The primary lesions are in the pulmonary artery and lung parenchyma
- The microfilaria may cause a pneumonitis and glomerulonephritis, and occasionally end up in unusual sites, e.g. anterior chamber of the eye, systemic arteries
- Infection with *Dirofilaria immitis* has been categorised into four presentations:
  (1) Asymptomatic cases

(2) Verminous pneumonitis
(3) Advanced heartworm disease with cor pulmonale
(4) Caval syndrome

CLINICAL FEATURES

- Many dogs remain asymptomatic
- The more common presentations include lethargy, loss of condition, exercise intolerance, breathlessness and cough
- Non-specific signs, such as vague illness, exercise intolerance, weight loss can occur
- Signs of right-sided congestive failure with *cor pulmonale* and marked ascites
- Sudden death
- Signs of forward heart failure
- Increased respiratory sounds
- There may be a prominent split second heart sound on auscultation and there may be a murmur of tricuspid regurgitation
- Dogs with the caval syndrome may have more advanced signs of forward and backward right-sided heart failure, with jaundice and slightly dark urine (haemoglobinuria)

DIAGNOSIS

Clinical pathology
- Peripheral eosinophilia and basophilia
- The presence of microfilariae in the peripheral blood (60–95% of cases) is diagnostic

Note: Differentiation from the non-pathogenic worm *Dipetalonema reconditum* is essential

- Positive modified Knott test (filtration method)

- ELISA antigen tests detect mature female worms
- Serological testing (e.g. indirect fluorescent antibody test, IFA, and ELISA-based tests) not of value in *screening*, but valuable in supporting a diagnosis in dogs suspected of dirofilariasis

Radiography

Radiography is useful for evaluating the severity of the disease and for providing a prognosis.

- Tortuosity and 'pruning' of the whole of the lobar artery in severely affected cases
- Right-sided heart enlargement
- Pulmonary infiltrates with a mixed alveolar/interstitial pattern
- Radiographs can also be used to assess response to treatment: persistence of changes 6–12 months after treatment suggests continual infection

Echocardiography

- Right ventricular dilation and hypertrophy, and paradoxical septal wall motion
- Echodensities may be apparent in the right ventricular lumen, particularly with the caval syndrome

THERAPY

The reader should consult detailed textbooks for treatment protocols.

- *Asymptomatic dogs* showing minimal signs on radiography
  - The adulticide *sodium thiacetarsemide*
  - Be aware of potential side effects
    - phlebitis, anorexia, vomiting, depression, hepatotoxicity and thromboembolism
- *Severely affected* animals
  - Additional therapy prior to the use of adulticidal drugs
    - Glucocorticosteroids to control the pulmonary hypersensitivity problems (see PIE, pp. 158–9)
    - Therapy to control signs of congestive heart failure
- *Emergency caval syndrome* case
  - Direct surgical removal of the worms with long grasping forceps
- *Microfilariaemia*
  - Dithiazanine, levamisole or ivermectin
- *Prevention*
  - Avermectin (monthly) during mosquito season in enzootic areas

PROGNOSIS

Pulmonary thrombosis and DIC are possible complications, although the likelihood of these developing can be minimised by pre-treatment with aspirin. Asymptomatic and PIE cases (without granulomatosis) have a reasonably good prognosis, while advanced heartworm disease warrants a guarded prognosis and the caval syndrome carries a poor prognosis.

15 SYSTEMIC AND PULMONARY HYPERTENSION

SYSTEMIC HYPERTENSION

Hypertension is defined as arterial blood pressure increased above accepted normal levels and consistently elevated on repeated measurements at different times, in a non-stressed animal (Table 15.1).

MEASUREMENT

There is variation in blood pressure with fear, excitement or pain.

Direct
- By cannulation of an artery (e.g. femoral, metatarsal)
- Fairly invasive for routine clinical use, often used by anaesthesiologists

Indirect
- *Doppler* technique
  - Blood flow can be measured with a small Doppler ultrasound transducer located over a palpable artery, e.g. metacarpal artery
  - Cuff inflated proximal to the artery, i.e. above the carpus
  - Systolic blood pressure only
- *Oscillometric* technique
  - Detects the small changes in cuff pressure by the pulse
  - Useful in animals >10 kg body weight
  - Difficult to use reliably in the cat and toy breed dogs
  - Systolic and diastolic blood pressure, but diastolic measurements can be unreliable
- In both the Doppler and oscillometric techniques the cuff width should be approximately 40% of the limb circumference
- Measurements should be repeated at least five times and provide a consistent result

CLASSIFICATION OF SYSTEMIC HYPERTENSION

- *Primary* (or essential) – most common form in man and considered rare in small animals
- *Secondary* – more common form in small animals, with a number of possible causes
  - Renal disease

Table 15.1 Approximate criteria for normal and hypertensive systolic blood pressure

Breed	Normal (mmHg)	Hypertensive (mmHg)
Dog	100–140	>160–180
Sight Hounds	140–150	
Cat	110–150	>180–200

Note: Sight hounds tend to have slightly higher than average systolic blood pressure

○ Hyperthyroidism (cats)
○ Hyperadrenocorticism
○ Diabetes mellitus
○ Hyperaldosteronism
○ Polycythaemia
○ Hypothyroidism (dogs)
○ Phaeochromocytoma
○ Hyperoestrogenism
○ Acromegaly
○ Hyperparathyroidism and hyper-calcaemia

AETIOLOGY

The most common causes of hypertension are:
• Dog
  ○ Renal disease
  ○ Hyperadrenocorticism
• Cat
  ○ Renal disease
  ○ Hyperthyroidism
• Most dogs and cats with renal disease are believed to be hypertensive

CLINICAL FINDINGS

Common presenting signs
• Polydipsia and polyuria
• Ocular signs
  ○ Acute blindness
  ○ Hyphaema
  ○ Retinal detachment, ischaemia, degeneration
  ○ Tortuosity of retinal vessels, perivascular blood leakage
  ○ Intraocular haemorrhage
  ○ Glaucoma
• Neurological signs
  ○ Ataxia
  ○ Seizures
  ○ Dementia
  ○ Coma
• Dyspnoea
• Inappetance

• Lethargy
• Cardiac signs
  ○ Systolic murmur
  ○ Gallop sounds
  ○ Left ventricular concentric hypertrophy

In the kidneys, a persistent increase in glomerular pressure results in glomerulosclerosis and loss of functional nephrons. This may lead to proteinuria and elevated blood urea and creatinine.

THERAPY

• Treatment should be directed towards the underlying cause
• Weight control is important in obese animals
• Sodium restriction may help in mild hypertension
• The drug which is currently recommended as first choice in cats is *amlodipine*, and it may be finding increasing use in dogs as well

---

Dose of amlodipine
Cats　0.625–1.25 mg per cat sid
Dogs　Starting dose of 0.05 mg/kg bid increasing to effect to a maximum of 0.1 mg/kg bid

---

• When there is renal failure, especially with protein loss, an ACE inhibitor is considered beneficial
• The urine protein:creatinine ratio can be used to estimate protein loss
  ○ Significant >1.0
  ○ Suspicious 0.4–1.0
• Other drug options are: diltiazem, prazosin, β-blockers (atenolol or propranolol)
• Combinations of drugs are used when there is a poor response to a single drug
• Blood pressure should be reassessed weekly until satisfactory control is achieved; thereafter every 3–6 months

- Clinical pathology (particularly urea and creatinine) of any concurrent/ underlying medical condition should be monitored regularly

PROGNOSIS

The outlook for these patients depends on the underlying disease.

PULMONARY HYPERTENSION

Secondary pulmonary hypertension (i.e. due to other causes) is not uncommon in dogs, but rare in cats. As it is difficult to diagnose, it is likely to be under-diagnosed ante mortem. Primary pulmonary hypertension is considered rare in animals.

Normal pulmonary arterial pressure
- Systolic 15–25 mmHg
- Diastolic 5–10 mmHg

AETIOLOGY

Increased pulmonary vascular resistance
- Pulmonary embolism
  - Parasitic disease: heartworm, angiostrongylosis
  - Neoplasia (lymphosarcoma, bronchoalveolar carcinoma, pancreatic carcinoma, mammary gland carcinoma)
  - Systemic bacterial disease (sepsis)
  - Autoimmune haemolytic anaemia
  - Long-term, indwelling i/v catheter
  - Disseminated intravascular coagulation
  - Hyperadrenocorticism
  - Glomerular disease
  - Pancreatitis
  - Nephrotic syndrome
  - Diabetes mellitus
  - Right heart disease
- *Cor pulmonale* due to severe parenchymal lung disease
  - Idiopathic pulmonary fibrosis, particularly West Highland White Terriers
- High altitude disease
- Polycythaemia (>55%), such as is caused by chronic hypoxia

Increased pulmonary venous pressure, such as that caused by left heart failure
This usually causes only mild to moderate increase in pulmonary artery pressure (<50 mmHg)

Increased right ventricular cardiac output
- Left-to-right cardiac shunts
- In reversed shunts, pulmonary artery pressure will equate to aortic pressure (Eisenmenger's syndrome)
  - PDA
  - VSD
  - ASD

Cor pulmonale
The term *cor pulmonale* refers to the effects on the right heart of pulmonary hypertension caused by lung disease. Chronic pulmonary hypertension leads to *concentric hypertrophy* of the right ventricle. Acute pulmonary hypertension leads to *dilation* of the right ventricle. If there is tricuspid valve incompetence this may progress to right-sided congestive heart failure (e.g. ascites). Reduced right ventricular cardiac output can also lead to systemic forward failure.

DIAGNOSIS

Suspicion is raised by:

- Presenting clinical signs and history (see later)
- Presence of disease known to lead to pulmonary hypertension

Thoracic radiographs

- Interstitial/alveolar infiltrates
- Regional hyperlucency
- Pulmonary vascular changes
- Pulmonary artery bulge
- Arterial blunting
- Cardiomegaly
- Pleural effusion

Echocardiographic examination

- Right ventricular hypertrophy or dilation
- Right atrial enlargement
- Pulmonary artery bulge

Abdominal ultrasound

- Hepatomegaly
- Hepatic venous congestion
- Ascites

Doppler echocardiographic studies

- Valvular regurgitant jet velocities significantly higher than normal

---

Normal valve regurgitant velocities in the right heart, derived by Doppler studies

Normal pulmonary artery to right ventricular pressures

- Pulmonic regurgitant jet velocity of ~2.2 m/s

Normal right ventricular to right atrial pressures

- Tricuspid regurgitant jet velocity of ~2.8 m/s

Pulmonary hypertension classified by tricuspid valve pressure gradient

Mild	< 50 mmHg
Moderate	50–75 mmHg
Severe	>75 mmHg

Blood gas analysis

Arterial blood gases are abnormal in most cases (>80%), characterised by hypoxaemia, increased alveolar-arterial gradient and hypocapnia.

Cardiac catheterisation and scintigraphy

These are specialist centre techniques.

CLINICAL SIGNS

Clinical signs are often due to the primary cause of the hypertension. Signs of pulmonary hypertension are more marked following exertion while mild to moderate hypertension itself may not produce clinical signs.

Signs of severe pulmonary hypertension

- Dyspnoea >90% of cases
  - Often on exertion
  - +/– cyanosis
- Exercise intolerance
- Exertional fatigue
- Weakness or collapse/syncope on exertion
- Ascites

THERAPY

- Directed towards the underlying condition
- Oxygen supplementation
- Pulmonary vasodilators may be of some help, but most also cause systemic

hypotension leading to weakness or collapse; proof of their efficacy is lacking
  ○ Diltiazem
  ○ Amlodipine
  ○ ACE inhibitors
  ○ Hydralazine
  ○ Sildenafil
  ○ Pimobendan
  ○ Bosentan
• Anticoagulant drugs
  ○ If pulmonary emboli are suspected
  ○ Inherent fibrinolysis will also assist in resolution of acute emboli
  ○ Thrombolytics – limited veterinary data on their usefulness
    – Streptokinase
    – Urokinase
    – Tissue plasminogen activator

Aspirin
• Dogs: 5 mg/kg daily
• Cats: 5–30 mg twice a week

Heparin
• Loading dose 220 iu/kg i/v or s/c
• Low molecular weight heparins
  ○ Enoxaparin: Dog and cat: 1 mg/kg s/c bid
  ○ Dalteparin: Dog and cat: 100–200 iu/kg s/c bid

PROGNOSIS

Prognosis is poor to grave in most instances. Mortality rates are very high, but spontaneous resolution can occur, and patients that survive the initial acute phase can recover with appropriate therapy.

DISEASES OF THE
CARDIORESPIRATORY SYSTEM

16 DISEASES OF THE UPPER RESPIRATORY TRACT

RHINITIS

Rhinitis is an all-encompassing term describing a condition in which there is an active inflammatory reaction in the nasal passages causing sneezing, nasal discharge and nasal discomfort. Typically, it involves secondary bacterial infections that can be so deep-seated as to involve the adjacent bony structures. Where the condition results in chronic hyperplastic changes in the nasal mucosa, *chronic rhinitis* exists. This is often associated with *lymphocyte* and *plasma cell* infiltration. Rhinitis has a multiplicity of possible causes and each cause will have subtle differences regarding clinical signs, progression and treatment.

AETIOLOGY

Viral/rickettsial/bacterial
- Feline upper respiratory tract infections
  ○ Feline rhinotracheitis (herpes) virus (FRV)
  ○ Feline calici virus (FCV)
  ○ *Chlamydophila*
  ○ Reovirus
- *Bordetella bronchiseptica, Staphylococcus* and non-haemolytic *Streptococcus* spp and *Mycoplasma* spp
- Concurrent infection (FeLV, FIV)
- Stressful environments/opportunity for transmission of infectious agents
  ○ Catteries
  ○ Veterinary surgeries
  ○ Fomites
- Close contact between cats

Fungal
- *Aspergillus fumigatus* (dogs)
- *Cryptococcus neoformans*

Allergic
- Eosinophilic rhinitis
- Lymphoplasmacytic rhinitis

Neoplastic
- Most tumours develop in the caudal nasopharynx
- Up to 35% have secondary fungal infection
  ○ Rhinarial tumours
  ○ Fibrosarcomas, melanoma, and squamous cell carcinoma (cats)
  ○ Nasal cavity tumours
    – Benign nasopharyngeal polyps
    – Adenocarcinomas (most common)
    – Undifferentiated carcinomas
    – Squamous cell carcinomas
    – Fibrosarcomas
    – Mesenchymal tumours (relatively rare)
    – Lymphomas (both in FeLV+ and FeLV- cats)

Parasitic (specific geographic locations)
- *Pneumonyssoides caninum*
- *Linguatala serrata*

Anatomical defects
- Cleft palate
- Oronasal fistulas (dental disease)

Other causes

- Chronic hyperplastic rhinitis
- Foreign body reactions

CLINICAL FEATURES

- Nasal discharge
  - Unilateral/bilateral
  - Clear (serous) mucoid, mucopurulent or blood-tinged
- Sneezing
- Epistaxis
  - Neoplasia, foreign bodies
- Nasal stertor, gagging, choking (coughing)
- Facial deformity, facial pain
- Depigmentation around nares is often seen with aspergillosis
- Epiphora
- Conjunctivitis, buccal ulceration and stomatitis
  - Viral infections, *Chlamydophila*
- Pyrexia and lethargy, inappetance
  - Viral infections

DIAGNOSIS

- Agent isolation from nasal and ocular material
- Serological tests may be supportive of a diagnosis – beware of false negative results with aspergillosis

Radiography

- Turbinate lucency (neoplasia, *Aspergillus*)
- Increased soft tissue densities
- Perforation of the nasal septum
- Destruction of the nasal bones

Rhinoscopy

- Fungal plaques
- Visible masses
- Turbinate atrophy
- Mucopurulent material

Nasal sampling

- Biopsy samples
- Nasal washes
- Culture
- Visible fungal hyphae

THERAPY

- Rhinarial tumours
  - Excision, cryosurgery and radiotherapy
- Nasal cavity tumours
  - Rhinotomy, tumour excision, nasal curettage (palliative)
    - Ineffective on its own
  - Radiotherapy
    - Orthovoltage radiation after cyto-reductive surgery gives good survival
  - Chemotherapy
    - May be beneficial but has not yet been fully evaluated
- *Chlamydophila* infection
  - Tetracycline antibiotic (doxycycline)
- Viral infections
  - Preventative control with vaccination and good husbandry practice in catteries, and breeding colonies
  - Good nursing care
  - Nasal decongestants (steam inhalation)
  - Antibiotics for secondary bacterial infections
  - Anti-viral agents (trifluridine) for corneal ulcers (herpes virus)
  - Recombinant feline interferon (unproven efficacy)
- Feeding
  - Liquidised foods
  - Nasogastric or oesophagotomy feeding in chronic anorexia
  - Appetite stimulants (cyproheptadine, diazepam)
- Fungal infection – check for underlying immunosuppression or neoplasia
  - Surgical (topical application)
    - Instillation of fungicidal agents
    - One hour infusion of clotrimazole under general anaesthesia: 70%

success after one treatment, 90% success after two
- Enilconazole at 10 mg/kg q12hr for 14 days via indweling catheters
  ○ Medical (systemic administration)
    - Oral ketoconazole or fluconazole – 50–65% success
    - Oral itraconazole – 70% success
  ○ *Aspergillus* titres remain elevated for years after treatment
- Bacterial rhinitis
  ○ Clindamycin or cephalosporins most effective
- Allergic, eosinophilic, lymphocytic, plasmacytic rhinitis
  ○ Glucocorticosteroids
  ○ Azathioprine, cyclophosphamide in difficult or refractory cases

PROGNOSIS

- Viral infection
  ○ Recovery within 2–3 weeks
  ○ Persistent or recurrent URTI signs
  ○ Chronic upper respiratory tract signs requiring continuous conservative management
- Bacterial rhinitis
  ○ Cure with appropriate antibiotics
  ○ Can prove difficult to control
- Neoplasia
  ○ Palliative control
- Fungal rhinitis
  ○ Cure rate reasonably high with proper treatment

BRACHYCEPHALIC UPPER AIRWAY SYNDROME

A complex group of anatomical deformities, affecting several (brachycephalic) breeds, that result in varying degrees of upper airway obstruction.

AETIOLOGY

Congenital anatomical deformities (singly or in combination)
- Stenotic nares
- Extended/thickened soft palate
- Laryngeal deformities
- Laryngeal collapse
- Everted saccules
- Hypoplastic trachea

CLINICAL FEATURES

Signs of upper airway obstruction:
- Dyspnoea
- Inspiratory stridor
- Cyanosis

- Collapsing
- Exercise intolerance
- Worse on excitement, exercise and in a warm environment
- Signs of secondary complications
  ○ Aspiration pneumonia
  ○ Non-cardiogenic pulmonary oedema
  ○ Chronic bronchitis
  ○ Chronic pulmonary interstitial disease (lung fibrosis might be present, but this is not proven)
  ○ Aerophagia and gastric dilation
  ○ Sleep apnoea in Bulldogs
- Evidence of cardiac impairment may be difficult to obtain, but some animals may have pulmonary hypertension

DIAGNOSIS

Diagnosis is based on the typical brachycephalic breed with pronounced inspiratory stridor.

Radiography
- Thickened/extended soft palate
- *Cor pulmonale*
  - Right-sided heart enlargement
  - Hepatomegaly
- Hypoplastic trachea

Laryngoscopy/bronchoscopy
Visible anatomic deformity.

Electrocardiography
- P-pulmonale (tall P waves)
- Exaggerated respiratory sinus arrhythmia

THERAPY

- Surgical correction of operable anatomical abnormalities
  - Stenotic nares
  - Extended soft palate
  - Everted laryngeal saccules
  - Emergency/permanent tracheostomy
- Oxygen supplementation during crises
- Glucocorticosteroids to control laryngeal oedema
- Cage rest and exercise restriction
- Avoidance of exacerbating causes
  - Exercise
  - Excitement
  - Hot weather

PROGNOSIS

Fair prognosis if not too adversely affected, but poor to grave if seriously affected and not operatively correctable. A good outcome following surgery in Bulldogs is achieved in ~60% of dogs with a post-operative mortality rate of 14% (primarily from aspiration pneumonia).

LARYNGEAL PARALYSIS

Laryngeal paralysis is a failure to abduct the arytenoid cartilages during inspiration and is very common in geriatric dogs, particularly Labrador Retrievers.

- Labrador
- English Setter
- Trauma or damage to the recurrent laryngeal nerve

AETIOLOGY

- Idiopathic (most common)
  - Labrador Retrievers, Setters, large breeds
  - Geriatric dogs
- Polyneuropathies and myopathies
- Neuromuscular disease
  - Myasthenia gravis
- Congenital
  - Bouvier des Flandres
  - Siberian Husky
  - White-coated German Shepherds
  - Dalmation
  - English Bull Terrier
  - Rottweiler

CLINICAL SIGNS

- May not be apparent in milder cases until respiratory work increases
- Hyperthermia may exacerbate dyspnoea
- Inspiratory dyspnoea (stridor)
  - Progressive appearance over months or years
  - Exacerbated by excitement, exercise, stress and anxiety
  - Severe respiratory distress
- Exercise intolerance
- Cyanosis
- Collapse
- Muscle atrophy
- Neurological signs

- Dysphonia
- Coughing
  - Gagging, choking (laryngeal)
  - Coughing (secondary bronchial or lung)
- Non-cardiogenic pulmonary oedema
- Affected dogs are more prone to heat stroke

DIAGNOSIS

- Characteristic history
  - Large-breed dogs
  - Inspiratory dyspnoea
  - Can be exacerbated by digital pressure (pinching) of larynx
- Visualising failure of arytenoid abduction under light anaesthesia

THERAPY

- Sedation if distressed
- Oxygen supplementation
- Cage rest
- Cooling of hyperthermic dogs
- Glucocorticosteroids (laryngeal oedema)
- Laryngoplasty
  - Laryngeal tie-back (arytenoid lateralisation); 90% success rate

PROGNOSIS

Resolution with surgery should be expected, but the surgical correction may fail eventually. Overall outcome is good, but most cases are geriatric and prolonged survival cannot be expected. Poor prognosis if secondary aspiration bronchitis or pneumonia is present or if there is evidence of concurrent dysphagia.

LARYNGEAL NEOPLASIA

Laryngeal neoplasms are extremely rare in the dog and cat, but if they occur they should result in signs typical of laryngeal disease (cough, dyspnoea, dysphonia).

17 DISEASES OF THE LOWER AIRWAYS

TRACHEAL COLLAPSE

The term *tracheal collapse* tends to imply an all-or-nothing effect. In the majority of cases, however, dorsoventral flattening of the trachea and flaccidity of the dorsal membrane are the major problems, and the trachea may only develop a partial collapse.

AETIOLOGY

- Unknown
- Congenital maldevelopment of the tracheal cartilages
- Age-related degeneration of the tracheal cartilage
- Obesity or other respiratory diseases that compromise tracheal mechanics in dogs where the trachea lacks structural rigidity and the dorsal membrane is flaccid and wide

CLINICAL FEATURES

- A problem of toy breeds (e.g. Yorkshire Terrier)
- Related to the severity of the collapse
- More severe form in young dogs
- Trachea may be easily compressed on manipulation
- Most commonly affects middle-aged dogs (less severe form)
- Coughing (goose-honk, seal-bark sound)
  - Aggravated by excitement, lead-pulling and airway inflammation
- Inspiratory dyspnoea (stridor) (severe disease)
- Expiratory dyspnoea
- Signs attributable to development of other respiratory diseases (e.g. chronic bronchitis)
- Concurrent obesity in middle-aged dogs

DIAGNOSIS

- Typical breed with a chronic cough
- Check for concurrent hyperadrenocorticism

Radiography
- Plain radiographs have a 60% diagnostic rate
- Inspiratory and expiratory views of whole trachea are required
- Collapse of the extrathoracic trachea (inspiratory), intrathoracic trachea (expiratory) or at the thoracic inlet
- Secondary airway, lung and cardiac changes

Fluoroscopy
Dynamic narrowing of the trachea.

Bronchoscopy
- Visualisation of collapse
- The most successful technique in achieving a diagnosis
- Surgical grading (I to IV)

THERAPY

- Surgical correction for severe life-threatening tracheal collapse (grade IV)
  - Extraluminal support rings
  - Intraluminal stents
- Control of obesity in older dogs – particularly important
- Use a harness rather than a dog collar
- Bronchodilators and glucocorticosteroids for secondary airway and lung changes

- Antibiotics and mucolytics for secondary bacterial infections
- Selective use of sedatives and antitussives

PROGNOSIS

- Good response to therapy (medical or surgical) suggests a favourable prognosis
- Progressive disease resulting in eventual respiratory failure or intractable coughing

ACUTE TRACHEOBRONCHITIS (KENNEL COUGH)

AETIOLOGY

- Infection with *Bordetella bronchiseptica*, canine parainfluenza virus (CPiV)
- Other viruses (CAV-2, CDV), *Mycoplasma*
- Inhalation of infected aerosolised sputum
- Close physical contact with oronasal secretions, fomites etc.
- History of the dog being in a suitably infective environment

CLINICAL SIGNS

- Cough
  - Acute onset
  - Mild to severe
  - Paroxysmal, dry, harsh and hacking
- Mild systemic signs of pyrexia, anorexia and lethargy
- Clinical sings develop within 3–10 days of suspected exposure

DIAGNOSIS

- Typical history and clinical presentation
- Spontaneous resolution or predictable response to antibacterial therapy

- Diagnostic techniques rarely applied to these cases

TREATMENT

- Likely to be self-limiting in most cases (up to three weeks duration)
- Antibacterial agents speed resolution
  - Potentiated sulphonamides, fluoroquinolones, doxycycline
- Antitussives to control excessive coughing
- Antibiotics and mucolytics for secondary bacterial infections
- Isolate from other susceptible dogs
- Avoid excessive exercise and dry, dusty and cold environments
- Prophylactic vaccination reduces chances of infection in high-risk environments

PROGNOSIS

- Spontaneous remission of clinical signs
- Can take up to three weeks in some dogs
- Bronchopneumonia may develop in some dogs, but this is rare
- Development of a chronic non-responsive cough (chronic tracheobronchial syndrome) in some cases

CHRONIC TRACHEOBRONCHIAL SYNDROME

An uncommon sequel to acute tracheo-bronchitis that results in chronic coughing, but the dogs are otherwise unaffected.

May resolve spontaneously but can take up to 18 months to do so. Antitussive medication can be used to ease the coughing.

CHRONIC BRONCHITIS

(See also Feline asthma)
Chronic bronchitis is defined as chronic bronchial inflammation associated with mucus hypersecretion. On histopathology, there should be evidence of airway-wall thickening, an increase in goblet cell numbers, an increase in mucous gland size and widespread loss of ciliated epithelium.

AETIOLOGY

- Not known in most instances
- Excessive production of mucus itself causes plugging of smaller airways, and further damage to the airways by providing a suitable environment for secondary bacterial infections
- Secondary to respiratory infections
- Secondary to other chronic respiratory diseases
- Airway damage by inhaled irritants and allergens
- Defective mucociliary clearance mechanism – *immotile cilia syndrome* (*ciliary dyskinesia*)

CLINICAL SIGNS

- Marked variability in the clinical presentation
- Condition is progressive and the airway changes irreversible
- Cough for at least two months
- Tachypnoea and dyspnoea in advanced disease
- Exercise intolerance

- Respiratory embarrassment at rest or with mild exertion
- Pyrexic, anorexic or inappetant and lethargic (during episodes of concurrent bronchopneumonia)
- Debility and cachexia (advanced disease)
- Increased respiratory sounds on auscultation
  ○ Wheezes and crackles
  ○ Muffled heart sounds
- *Cor pulmonale* and right-sided congestive failure can develop in chronic cases

DIAGNOSIS

Diagnosis is based on the clinical features of the disease.

Radiography
- Increased bronchial markings
- Bronchiectasis
- Evidence of long-standing respiratory disease (*cor pulmonale*, right-sided cardiac enlargement and hepatomegaly, interstitial fibrosis)

Bronchoscopy
- Roughened bronchial walls
- Blanched mucosa or mucosal inflammation with hyperaemia
- Excess airway mucus visible
- Bronchiectasis

Bronchial and bronchoalveolar lavage samples
- Large amounts of mucus
- Variable numbers of polymorphonuclear

leucocytes (neutrophils and/or eosinophils), macrophages and plasma cells
- Curschmann's spirals may be present
- Variable bacterial population (mainly Gram negative aerobes)

TREATMENT

- Treat the underlying cause where possible
- Weight control in obese animals
- Trial the dog on a variety of medications, selecting those to give the best response
- Vigorous antibacterial therapy if concurrent bacterial bronchopneumonia present
- Glucocorticosteroids
  - Oral prednisolone
  - Inhalation glucocorticosteroids
- Bronchodilators – β-agonists methylxanthines

- Antibiotics if there is secondary airway infection
- Mucolysis
  - Mucolytic agents
  - Inhaled steam or nebulised hypertonic saline
  - Chest percussion and physiotherapy
- Expectorant agents are of questionable value
- Antitussives are contraindicated
- Rest and exercise control

PROGNOSIS

- Depends on the initial response to therapy
- Recurrent conditions such as bronchopheumonia, that prove increasingly difficult to control
- Eventual deterioration and respiratory failure (months to years)

BRONCHIECTASIS

Usually a sequel to other severe and chronic respiratory diseases such as *chronic bronchitis, ciliary dyskinesia* and *eosinophilic bronchitis* (see also Chronic bronchitis, above).

DIAGNOSIS

Radiography
Cylindrical or saccular dilatation of lobar bronchi visible.

Bronchoscopy
Cavernous dilated airways, with roughened mucosa and accumulation of purulent exudates.

TREATMENT

- Management of the underlying cause
- Control of airway hygiene
- Control of 20 infections (bronchopneumonia)

AIRWAY FOREIGN BODIES

Inhalation of small objects is relatively uncommon, but inhalation of food material or, worse, gastric contents, is more common and more hazardous (see Pneumonia, pp. 154–6).

AETIOLOGY

- Discrete objects including grass-seed heads, small twigs and small stones
- Inhaled during playing, exercising etc.

- Hair, food and fluids
- Medications

CLINICAL SIGNS

- Sudden onset of clinical signs associated with severe distress and panic
- Coughing
  - Pronounced harsh and hacking with retching
  - Subsides after 3–4 days becoming soft and paroxysmal
  - Can persist for months
- Respiratory distress, depending on:
  - Size of the object
  - Location (rostral to carina if severe dyspnoea, but rare event)
- Marked halitosis after weeks to months
- Otherwise often normal

DIAGNOSIS

History of coughing after playing with an object or running through undergrowth etc.

Radiography
- Radiodense metal or stone objects
- Increased density in the hilar region
- Pleural effusion or lung consolidation with air bronchograms

Bronchoscopy
Visualisation of inhaled object.

THERAPY

- Remove as soon as possible
  - Bronchoscopic retrieval by experienced operator usually successful
  - Thoracotomy
    - Large objects occluding the trachea
    - Removal of consolidated lung lobe
    - Drain, debride and examine the pleural space
- Antibacterial therapy
  - Bronchopneumonia
  - Lung-lobe consolidation
  - Pyothorax

PROGNOSIS

Discrete small foreign bodies can be easily removed by bronchoscopy. Foreign body migration is rare but can cause lung abscessation and pleural contamination. Very large foreign bodies can occlude the airway causing asphyxia and death.

DISEASES OF THE
CARDIORESPIRATORY SYSTEM

18 DISEASES OF THE LUNG PARENCHYMA

PULMONARY THROMBOEMBOLISM (SEE CHAPTER 15, P. 41)

PNEUMONIA

Pneumonia is defined as inflammation of the lungs and can be classified based on:
- Anatomical location
  - Bronchopneumonia (inflammation involving alveoli and their associated airways)
  - Interstitial pneumonia
  - Lobar pneumonia
- Predominant cell type involved (e.g. eosinophilic pneumonia)
- Aetiology (e.g. aspiration pneumonia)
- Type of reaction in the lung (e.g. lipoid pneumonia)

AETIOLOGY

Infectious agents
Infectious agents are the most common causes of pneumonia in the cat and dog and several agents can be involved at the same time.

Viruses
Require secondary bacterial infections to cause significant disease
- Canine distemper virus (CDV)
- Canine adenovirus II (CAV-2)
- Parainfluenza virus
- Upper respiratory tract viruses in cats

Bacteria
Most are secondary pathogens and are part of the normal oral and respiratory flora.

- *Bordetella bronchiseptica* (PRIMARY)
- β-haemolytic *Streptococcus*
- *Pasteurella* spp
- *Klebsiella* and *Proteus* spp
- *Escherichia coli* and other Gram negative organisms
- *Mycoplasma* agents

Microaerophilic organisms
Actinomyces and *Nocardia* spp.

> **Note:** Deciding whether or not an isolated organism is significant is qualitative. Heavy growths of any of the organisms listed above suggest involvement in the disease process.

Fungi
Fungi are restricted to specific geographical areas.
- Histoplasmosis
- Blastomycosis
- Coccidiomycosis
- Cryptococcosis
- Aspergillosis

Predisposing diseases and causes
Several diseases and scenarios predispose to the development of pneumonia and secondary bacterial proliferation. Resident bacterial flora proliferate in response to respiratory system insult.

- Chronic bronchitis
- Immotile cilia syndrome
- Acute tracheobronchitis
- Laryngeal paralysis
- Smoke inhalation
- Inhaled food and fluids
- Oral dosing with medications
- Cleft palate
- Swallowing defects
- Megaoesophagus
- Discrete foreign bodies
- Inhaled allergens (eosinophilic pneumonia)
- Airway and lung parasites
- Endogenous and exogenous toxins
- Acquired or inherited immunodeficiency syndromes
- Protozoal infections (toxoplasmosis, pneumocystosis, neosporosis)

CLINICAL SIGNS

Clinical signs are variable depending on the extent of lung involvement, and can vary from acute to chronic and mild to severe.

- Coughing (soft and non-productive)
- Dyspnoea and tachypnoea (severe bronchopneumonia)
- Tachypnoea at rest or after mild exercise or exertion
- Systemic signs (pyrexia, lethargy, anorexia and cachexia)
- Often afebrile
- Signs of concurrent systemic or multisystem disease
  - Swallowing defects, oesophageal and gastrointestinal disorders (aspiration pneumonia)
- Recent anaesthesia, hospitalisation immunosuppression

DIAGNOSIS

Clinical history and clinical signs are very useful in making a diagnosis. Severe forms of bronchopneumonia are usually acute in onset.

Haematology and biochemistry

- Leucocytosis – neutrophilia, with or without a left shift, may be found in some cases
- May have a normal leucogram
- Circulating eosinophilia (allergic or parasitic pneumonia)
- Biochemical changes are non-specific and non-diagnostic

Radiography

Crucial to diagnosis, but changes may not always correlate with the severity of clinical signs.

- Localised dense areas of consolidation (lobar pneumonia)
- Diffuse interstitial patterns
- Alveolar pattern with air bronchograms (classic description), diffuse or localised
- Cranioventral distribution common

Bronchoscopy

Beneficial to diagnosis, but only if patient can tolerate an anaesthetic.

- Inflammatory exudates in the airways
- Mucopurulent material exiting single lobar bronchus
- Location of changes often correlates with radiographic findings

Airway sampling and bronchoalveolar lavage

- Collection of material for cytology and culture
- Large numbers of inflammatory cells are usually recovered
- The predominant cell types are neutrophils and macrophages
- Eosinophils suggest an allergic or parasitic cause

Culture and sensitivity testing

- Not always successful and the delay in obtaining culture results is a problem

- Heavy growth is an important consideration, but anaerobic organisms can take up to six weeks to identify
- Gram negative bacteria most common
- Identification of the culprit pathogens improves treatment success

THERAPY

Vigorous and sustained therapy is required for severe acute bacterial bronchopneumonia.

- Antibacterial therapy (except for eosinophilic pneumonias)
  - Preferably based on culture and sensitivity results
  - Necessary for between 4–12 weeks
  - Empirical antibiotic selection more common
    - Potentiated sulphonamides at 30 mg/kg q12hr
  - Antibacterial agents with broad spectrum activity that penetrate well into lung tissue
  - Target Gram negative aerobes (e.g. fluoroquinolones), but may also have to target anaerobes (e.g. clindamycin)
  - Combination therapy may also be used in particularly difficult cases
- Oxygen supplementation (if SPO_2 less than 90%) – humidification essential and avoid excessive supplementation
- Monitor arterial O_2 daily if possible to assess response to therapy

- Good nursing care, cage rest and warmth, supportive nutrition and fluid therapy
- Bronchodilators and mucolytics of debatable benefit
- Physiotherapy to assist removal of mucopurulent material from the airways
  - Chest percussion and coupage
  - Inhalation of steam or nebulised saline
  - Expectorant agents are ineffective and antitussives should never be used
  - Encourage mild exercise (walking) in less severe cases
- Anti-inflammatory agents can be used to control pyrexia
- Glucocorticosteroids in eosinophilic pneumonia
- Surgical removal of chronically damaged/infected lung lobes
- Anti-fungal therapy against specific agents in enzootic areas

PROGNOSIS

Clinical outcome will depend on the rapidity and intensity of therapy, and the success in treating non-respiratory underlying problems. Severe acute bronchopneumonia can be cured. Recurrent aspiration pneumonia carries a particularly poor prognosis. Failure to control pneumonia can result in death, chronic bronchopneumonia, chronic interstitial and alveolar fibrosis, *cor pulmonale* or pulmonary abscessation.

RESPIRATORY FUNGAL DISEASES

Pulmonary involvement with fungal agents tends to have a reasonably strict geographical distribution, and fungal pneumonia is not readily recognised in the British Isles. They are particularly prevalent in the mid-western United States and Australia. Fungal pneumonias can occur in both dogs and cats.

AETIOLOGY

- *Histoplasma capsulatum*, *Coccidioides immitis*, *Blastomyces dermatitidis* (North America), *Aspergillus fumigatus* (Western Australia, possibly worldwide) and *Cryptococcus* (worldwide) cause mycotic pneumonias

- *Aspergillus fumigatus* causes nasal disease worldwide

CLINICAL FEATURES

- Localised, mild, sub-clinical or severe pulmonary disease or systemic infection
- Clinical signs depend on the degree of systemic involvement

Histoplasmosis
- Transient pyrexia and coughing with resolution, or
- Development of severe pulmonary disease with coughing, dyspnoea, tachypnoea, inappetance and cachexia, or
- Insidious development of clinical signs may occur with granulomatous interstitial pneumonia and hilar lymphadenopathy, causing chronic coughing

Blastomycosis
- Similar to histoplasmosis, but can be rapidly fatal
- Hilar lymphadenopathy is less likely and more common in young, male large-breed dogs

Coccidiomycosis
- Mild to severe respiratory disease or fatal multi-system involvement
- Noted more in young, male, large-breed dogs

DIAGNOSIS

Appropriate clinical signs in animals from enzootic areas.

Radiography
Changes can vary widely and include:
- Hilar lymphadenopathy
- Nodular interstitial patterns
- Increased bronchial markings and alveolar patterns

- Some inactive lesions may become calcified

Bronchial samples
- Agent isolation from bronchial samples and transthoracic needle samples and biopsies of peripheral lymph nodes
- Culture can be performed, but only in specialist laboratories, to avoid accidental infection of personnel

Serological tests
- Useful for cryptococcosis and coccidiomycosis, but less useful for other fungal infections
- False negative results are common for histoplasmosis.

TREATMENT

- The mainstay of treatment is anti-fungal agents: amphotericin B, ketoconazole, itraconazole, either alone or in combination with each other
- Medication may have to be continued for several months, and the potential drug side effects must be appreciated
- The use of the antimetabolite flucytosine, and the chitin inhibitors nikkomycin and lufenuron, are still being evaluated
- Histoplasmosis may resolve spontaneously, but the danger of dissemination makes treatment necessary and ketoconcazole alone can be sufficient
- Success with treatment of Blastomycosis is reported as being 60–70%

For more detailed guidelines on the treatment of pulmonary mycotic diseases consult relevant monographs and textbooks.

PROGNOSIS

The outcome is usually favourable with the correct treatment.

PULMONARY INFILTRATION WITH EOSINOPHILS (EOSINOPHILIA) (PIE)

(See also Feline asthma syndrome, below)

This is a clinical syndrome characterised by eosinophil infiltration into the respiratory system. It can cause clinical disease dependent on the intensity of the eosinophilic reaction and in what part of the respiratory system the eosinophils accumulate.

AETIOLOGY

- Helminth parasites
- Migrating ascarid larvae
- *Aelurostrongylus abstrusus* (cat)
- *Oslerus osleri* and *Crenosoma vulpis* (dog)
- *Angiostrongylus vasorum*
- *Dirofilaria immitis* (eosinophilic granulomas)
- Type I immediate hypersensitivity (possibly inhaled allergens) (see Feline asthma syndrome)
- Unknown

CLINICAL FEATURES (PIE)

- Marked variability (depending on degree of airway and/or lung involvement)
- Cough
- Dyspnoea and tachypnoea
- Exercise intolerance
- Usually otherwise clinically normal
- Usually bright, alert and non-febrile

DIAGNOSIS

- Significant numbers of eosinophils in airway or lung samples
- Circulating eosinophilia supports a diagnosis

- Occasional circulating basophilia (rare but significant: suspect pulmonary eosinophilic granuloma as this is most commonly seen in *Dirofilaria immitis* enzootic areas)

Radiography

- Variable, mild to severe bronchial, interstitial and alveolar patterns
- A pure diffuse interstitial pattern would be highly suspicious for PIE

Bronchoscopy

- Non-specific and variable
- Increased amounts of mucus
- Rarely significant airway mucosal changes

TREATMENT

- Important to treat for parasitism (seven days course of fenbendazole)
- Glucocorticosteroids
  - Rapid resolution of the clinical signs
  - Emergency therapy may be required (i/v methylprednisolone succinate or dexamethasone)
  - Oral prednisolone therapy
    - 1 mg/kg q24h reducing to 0.2 mg/kg q48h, maintained for two months
  - Long-term continuous therapy maybe required
  - Delivery by inhalation might be worth attempting to reduce glucocorticosteroid side effects
- Supplement with azathioprine in rare refractory cases
- Avoidance of allergens should be attempted if possible

PROGNOSIS

- Good to excellent in most cases

- Occasionally may need life-long (continuous, but more usually intermittent) therapy

FELINE ASTHMA SYNDROME

(See also PIE)
Asthma can be defined as a reversible form of bronchoconstriction that results in wheezing and dyspnoea, but which also involves a significant inflammatory component.

AETIOLOGY

- Possibly involving Type I or Type III hypersensitivity reactions
- Airway hypersensitivity reaction to inhaled allergens
  - House dust mites
  - Air pollution
  - Smoke
  - Carpet cleaners
  - Aair fresheners and deodorants/sprays
  - Seasonal pollens
  - Respiratory infections
  - Others unknown

CLINICAL FEATURES

- Variable severity, often paroxysmal
- Coughing
- Expiratory wheezing
- Pulmonary crackles
- Dyspnoea and tachypnoea
- Orthopnoea
- Rib fractures +/− pneumothorax

Note: Chronic coughing is the single most common clinical sign with asthma, however to many owners this can seem like retching or even vomiting. Cats with cardiomegaly or heart failure rarely cough.

DIAGNOSIS

- History and clinical signs
- Young to middle-aged cats more commonly affected, with Siamese over-represented
- Eosinophils in airway samples
  - Common in some normal cats
  - Maybe non-degenerate neutrophil-rich airway sample

Radiography
- Predominantly a bronchial pattern
- However the pattern can be mixed
- Hyperinflation (air-trapping), hyperlucency of the lung field, with flattening of the diaphragm
- Collapse of middle or cranial lung lobe is not uncommon (more often the right middle lung lobe)

Haematology
Circulating eosinophilia in 20% of cases.

Note: A rapid response to dexamethasone, bronchodilators and oxygen is highly suggestive of a diagnosis of asthma in cats.

THERAPY

- Treatment depends on the severity and the persistence of clinical signs
- Exclusion from the owner's bedroom (human dander and house dust mite)
- Removal of potential triggers, e.g. household aerosol products, cat litter dust etc.

DISEASES OF THE CARDIORESPIRATORY SYSTEM

- Important to rule out parasitism, by appropriate treatment (e.g. seven days course of fenbendazole)
- Bronchodilators may be of some benefit
  - β-2-adrenoreceptor agonists
    - Terbutaline at 0.625–1.25 mg per cat q8–12h
    - Salbutamol or albuterol by inhalation (with Aerocat spacer device)
  - Methylxanthine agents (aminophyline)
- Glucocorticosteroids are the primary method of control
  - Oral
    - Prednisolone
    - 1–2 mg/kg q12h for 7–10 days then slowly reducing to 0.2 mg/kg q48h
  - By inhalation using a paediatric spacer device (Aerocat)
    - Fluticasone proprionate at 125 μg q12h
    - Beclomethasone proprionate 100 μg q12h
  - The response is usually rapid, but therapy should be continued for eight weeks and then withdrawn. If clinical signs recur shortly after cessation of therapy, continuous therapy will probably be necessary.

> **Note:** Under-treatment of asthma with steroids may lead to bronchiectasis – an irreversible airway condition with a grave prognosis.

- Severely affected cases require oxygen therapy, intravenous glucocorticosteroids and intravenous or nebulised/inhaled bronchodilators
- Oxygen enriched environment in acute-onset severely affected cats
- Other treatments, usually in conjunction with glucocorticosteroids or in an attempt to reduce steroid dose

  - Cyproheptadine (serotonin antagonist) – 0.1–0.5 mg/kg q8–12h po (prophylactric)
  - Cyclosporin might be indicated if there is irreversible airway disease
  - Leukotriene receptor antagonists have doubtful or unproven efficacy in the treatment of feline asthma, but may be of some benefit in some cases
- A covering antibiotic course is prudent, as 25% of cats with lower airway disease may also have *Mycoplasma* infections (doxycycline for 10–14 days)

> **Note:** Rapid reversal of profound bronchoconstriction is required in cats with *status asthmaticus*. Intravenous atropine (20–40 μg/kg) or adrenaline (20 μg/kg [1:10000 solution = 100 μg/ml]) i/m, i/v or s/c can be used once the potentially serious side effects (particularly arrhythmias with adrenaline) are understood. Terbutaline can also be used at 0.01 mg/kg i/v, i/m or s/c. Alternatively, the less hazardous intravenous administration of rapidly acting glucocorticosteroids, such as methylprednisolone succinate or dexamethasone (0.1–0.5 mg/kg i/v or i/m), can be undertaken. The cat must have a patent airway and supplemental oxygen should be available.

PROGNOSIS

Most cats respond favourably to oral prednisolone and can be controlled on an alternate-day, low-dose regime. Untreated cases may develop irreversible chronic bronchitis and irreversible lung changes.

IDIOPATHIC PULMONARY FIBROSIS

The exact mechanisms underlying the development of chronic interstitial fibrosis in dog and cat lung are not known. It is probable that these changes are secondary to other underlying respiratory and non-respiratory diseases. *Idiopathic pulmonary fibrosis* (IPF) is the most commonly recognised cause of this problem.

AETIOLOGY

- Idiopathic pulmonary fibrosis – West Highland White (WHWT) and Cairn Terriers
- Secondary to other chronic respiratory conditions
- Toxins (paraquat)
- Incidental radiographic finding

CLINICAL FEATURES (IPF IN WHWT)

- Develops slowly over months to years
- Dyspnoea and tachypnoea noted initially
- Exercise intolerance
- Inspiratory crackles
  - A cardinal feature of the disease
- Coughing
  - May appear at later stages of the disease
- Otherwise bright, alert, responsive with normal appetite

DIAGNOSIS

- Exclusion of all other possible causes (chronic bronchitis)
- Clinical history and development of clinical signs, particularly inspiratory crackles, in susceptible breeds

Radiography

- Generalised increase in interstitial density throughout the entire lung field
- *Cor pulmonale* with right-sided cardiomegaly and hepatomegaly (see Chapter 15)

Bronchoscopy

- Dynamic collapsing of lobar bronchi during expiration
- Lack of evidence of active or chronic airway inflammation (differentiation from *chronic bronchitis*)

Airway cytology

Normal or mild inflammatory profile; often a mild mucoid discharge

Lung pathology

- Required for definitive confirmation, but rarely obtained
- Pathological characteristics poorly described to date

High resolution computed tomography

- Patchy changes
- Ground-glass appearance
- Honeycombing
- Traction bronchiectasis
- Sub-pleural distribution of lesions

TREATMENT

- Variable response and invariably ineffective
- An initial good response would suggest chronic bronchitis is present or is contributing to the clinical presentation
- Glucocorticosteroids
  - Prednisolone at anti-inflammatory doses, reducing to the lowest possible dose, administered on alternate days

DISEASES OF THE CARDIORESPIRATORY SYSTEM

- Bronchodilators – theophylline, clenbuterol
- Azathioprine (with prednisolone)
- Obesity control and exercise restriction

Note: The effectiveness of antifibrotic agents, such as colchicine, in the treatment of IPF in dogs, is unproven and the evidence from human studies suggests such agents are ineffective.

PULMONARY NEOPLASIA

CLASSIFICATION (AETIOLOGY UNKNOWN)

Primary
- Adenocarcinoma (95%)
- Squamous cell and bronchogenic (columnar cell) carcinoma

Secondary (metastatic spread)
- Mammary and thyroidal adenocarcinoma
- Tonsillar carcinoma
- Digital melanoma
- Lymphosarcoma
- Osteosarcoma

Multicentric neoplasms
- Lymphoma

CLINICAL FEATURES

- Variable and progressive (weeks or months)
- Middle-aged to old animals
- Coughing (compression of larger airways)
- Dyspnoea and tachypnoea
- Expiratory dyspnoea (expiratory grunt)
- Exercise intolerance
- Haemoptysis
- Paraneoplastic signs

PROGNOSIS

Condition is progressive and respiratory failure occurs eventually. Survival time from diagnosis is approximately 6–12 months, but some individuals can survive up to three years.

- ○ Hypertrophic pulmonary osteopathy
- ○ Pyrexia
- ○ Anorexia and cachexia
- ○ General lethargy
- ○ Gastrointestinal signs
- ○ Secondary bronchopneumonia
- ○ Hypercalcaemia
- ○ Peripheral neuropathy or polymyositis
- Pneumothorax

DIAGNOSIS

Diagnosis is based on appropriate clinical history, signs and radiographic evidence.

Radiography
- Solitary masses
- Diffuse, single-lobe density
- Multiple, well-delineated masses
- Multiple, diffuse masses
- Mixed, diffuse, alveolar and interstitial patterns
- Pleural effusion
- Soft tissue densities less than 3 mm will not be visible on radiography

Ultrasonography
- Identifies mass lesions, particularly if obscured by pleural effusion
- Assists in biopsy sampling

Bronchoscopy

Dynamic compression of larger airways and the presence of blood-tinged mucus in the airway.

Airway cytology

Neoplastic cells may be be identified (definitive diagnosis).

Lung biopsy

- Transthoracic fine-needle biopsy (neoplastic cells in aspirate)
- Trucut biopsy of mass lesions adjacent to chest wall
- Thoracotomy biopsy
- Neoplastic cells in pleural effusion (rare finding)
- Identification of malignant neoplasm elsewhere in the body (metastatic disease)

TREATMENT

Primary lung tumour

- Surgical removal of operable masses

- Median survival times for dogs with primary lung tumours following complete surgical excision is 12 months (range 0–47 months), but for those with clinical signs the median survival time is eight months
- Early surgical intervention might improve survival
- Palliative medical therapy for inoperable cases (e.g. glucocorticosteroids)
- Chemotherapy and radiotherapy have not been evaluated in dogs and cats

Secondary neoplasia

- Surgery ill-advised
- Chemotherapy may be palliative, but there are no recommendations as to protocols

PROGNOSIS

- Poor to grave – eventual death due to disseminated pulmonary neoplasia
- Longer survival with early surgical intervention in primary neoplasia

ACUTE RESPIRATORY DISTRESS SYNDROME (ARDS)

Acute respiratory distress syndrome and *acute lung injury* are two clinical syndromes typified by an excessive response to lung injury that result in respiratory failure. They are clinical syndromes more likely to be seen in critically ill patients, and involve a complex pathogenesis of pulmonary oedema, inflammation and lung remodelling. Pulmonary hypertension is often a consequence of the lung damage.

AETIOLOGY

The underlying cause is not known, but the syndrome is precipitated by a number of risk factors:

- Pneumonia
- Pulmonary contusion
- Non-cardiogenic pulmonary oedema
- Sepsis
- Trauma
- Multi-system systemic illness

CLINICAL FEATURES

- Clinical signs due to the underlying risk factor
- Severe respiratory distress

DIAGNOSIS

- History of worsening respiratory function in a critically-ill patient
- Diffuse pulmonary infiltrates seen on radiography
- Diagnostic test results for the suspected risk factor

TREATMENT

- Treat the underlying cause (risk factor disease)

- Positive pressure ventilation (limited to very few specialist centres)
- Supportive care
  - Nutrition
  - Fluids
  - Antibacterial agents

PROGNOSIS

Very poor prognosis, with poor survival outcome if problem is recognised too late or vigorous treatment not instituted early enough or for sufficient length of time.

PULMONARY CONTUSION AND PULMONARY HAEMORRHAGE

Pulmonary contusion and haemorrhage can be considered together, as contusion mainly results in haemorrhage. In addition to pulmonary contusion, trauma can result in pneumothorax, fractured ribs and flail chest, haemothorax and diaphragmatic rupture.

AETIOLOGY

- Blunt trauma to the chest
  - Road traffic accidents
  - Blast injuries
- Other causes of bleeding
- Neoplasia
- Coagulopathies

CLINICAL FEATURES

- Respiratory distress in the context of chest trauma
  - Respiration usually laboured
  - Slow, purposeful inspiration and expiration
  - Expiratory dyspnoea with an obvious end-expiratory grunt
    - Breathing pattern is affected by the degree of pain
    - Respiratory signs might be mild
- Cardiac arrhythmias (traumatic myocarditis)
- Signs of trauma to the chest
  - Fractured ribs
  - Other fractures indicating trauma
  - Open wounds
  - Abrasions or oil or dirt marks on the coat
  - Flail-chest segments
- Respiratory signs can take 24–48 hours to develop and 7–10 days to resolve
- Pulmonary haemorrhage can be clinically similar to pneumonia

DIAGNOSIS

- History of blunt trauma
- Known exposure to rodenticides (haemorrhage)
- Abnormal coagulation profiles
- Arterial blood gas abnormalities

Radiography
- Consolidated lung area

- Diffuse alveolar infiltrates
- Fractured ribs
- Intrapulmonary haemorrhage
- Pneumothorax, haemothorax, pneumo-mediastinum
- Ruptured diaphragm

THERAPY

- Supportive care
  - Oxygen supplementation
  - Pain control (e.g. butorphanol)
- Surgical correction of flail chest and ruptured diaphragm
- Lung lobectomy should be considered if condition fails to resolve
- Pulmonary contusion should be allowed to resolve itself

- Use of glucocorticosteroids, antibacterial agents and diuretics is controversial and their efficacy unproven

PROGNOSIS

Prognosis depends on degree of lung damage and/or other thoracic damage. In some cases permanent lung consolidation may occur, but if there are no respiratory signs therapy is not required. Lung contusion and haemorrhage will resolve in due course, but permanent lung damage is possible. Death, if it occurs, often happens within the first four hours or in the 48–72 hour period after the traumatic event.

PULMONARY OEDEMA

Pulmonary oedema is mainly cardiogenic in cats and dogs, but may also be due to non-cardiogenic causes.

AETIOLOGY

Cardiogenic
Left-sided congestive failure (see Chapter 6).

Non-cardiogenic
- Increased vascular permeability
  - Hypoalbuminaemia
  - Inhalation of toxic substances and irritants
  - Ingestion of toxins (e.g. the agricultural weedkiller paraquat)
  - Anaphylactic reactions
  - Multi-systemic inflammatory and non-inflammatory diseases (e.g. uraemia, acute pancreatitis, sepsis)
  - Lung inflammation
- Severe upper airway obstruction

- Neurogenic
  - Severe epileptiform seizures
  - Electrocution
  - Cranial trauma

> **Note:** The general effect of several of these diseases is to cause so-called 'shock-lung' syndrome (Adult Respiratory Distress Syndrome).

CLINICAL FEATURES

- Varying degrees of respiratory distress
  - Tachypnoea, dyspnoea or orthopnoea
- Exercise intolerance
- Cough
- Cyanosis that is readily visible or easily elicited
- Oedema fluid can appear from the nostrils or from the mouth
- Harsh lung sounds with or without crackles

DISEASES OF THE CARDIORESPIRATORY SYSTEM

- Clinical signs related to the underlying aetiology

DIAGNOSIS

Suspicious history or clinical signs:
- Trauma
- Neurological disease
- Severe systemic illness (e.g. acute pancreatitis)
- Smoke inhalation
- Ingestion of toxins

Radiography
- Variable increased interstitial and/or alveolar pattern with or without air bronchograms
- Cardiomegaly
- Prominent distended pulmonary vessels

Biochemistry
Hypoalbuminaemia (less than 10–15 g/l).

Blood gas analysis
- Alveolar-arterial gradient increased
- Useful to assess respiratory function

TREATMENT

Cardiogenic pulmonary oedema
See treatment of Congestive heart failure, Chapter 6, pp. 66–70

Non-cardiogenic pulmonary oedema
- Treatment of the underlying cause
- Can resolve spontaneously
- Cage rest and minimise stress
- Diuretics and vasodilators are the mainstay of treatment of CHF and may be of benefit in the treatment of non-cardiogenic pulmonary oedema, although their efficacy may be debatable
- Supplemental oxygen therapy
- Sedation if the patient is particularly anxious

PROGNOSIS

Prognosis depends on severity and underlying cause. If the underlying cause can be resolved then the prognosis is good. However, severe pulmonary oedema may be uncontrollable and death may be inevitable.

CAVITARY LESIONS OF THE LUNGS

Cavitary lesions are relatively rare and are often detected incidentally. They may be congenital or acquired and contain:
- Air
- Serous fluid
- Blood
- Purulent material
- Sterile inflammatory material
- Necrotic material

Seven types of cavitary lesion are recognised in dogs and cats including:
(1) Cysts
(2) Bullae
(3) Blebs (sub-pleural, air-filled)
(4) Abscesses
(5) Cystic bronchiectasis (bronchial dilation)
(6) Pneumatocoeles
(7) Parasitic cysts

CLINICAL SIGNS

- Asymptomatic
- Pneumothorax and signs of acute respiratory distress (see Chapter 19, p. 171)
- Signs of chronic bronchial disease (bronchiectasis) and/or chronic bronchopneumonia

DIAGNOSIS

Radiography
- Ante mortem incidental finding
- Single or multiple delineated bullous lesions
- Pneumothorax (ruptured cyst)

THERAPY
- None if incidental and asymptomatic
- Treat the underlying cause or secondary complications
- Lung lobectomy
- Some may resolve spontaneously

EMPHYSEMA

Emphysema is rarely of clinical significance and is often an incidental finding on post mortem. Congenital lobar and bullous forms are described in young dogs. In acquired emphysema, changes are secondary to chronic respiratory diseases.

CLINICAL SIGNS

- Expiratory dyspnoea
- Inspiratory crackles
- Cyanosis may be present
- Signs of concurrent chronic bronchitis and bronchopneumonia

DIAGNOSIS

Diagnosis is by radiography demonstrating increased areas of lucency. Radiographic signs of chronic bronchitis and bronchopneumonia may mask the emphysematous pattern.

THERAPY

- Treat the underlying bronchitis and pneumonia
- Surgical removal of affected lung lobes (congenital forms)
- Acquired bullous lesions can often be left untreated

LUNG LOBE COLLAPSE AND TORSION

Relatively rare occurrence, particularly torsion. Collapse can occur for a variety of reasons.

AETIOLOGY

- A sequel to lung consolidation caused by airway obstruction, bronchopneumonia, other lung parenchymal diseases, pleural effusions, pneumothorax or atelectasis for any reason, including prolonged recumbency

- Spontaneous torsion occurs in certain predisposed, deep-chested breeds (e.g. Afghan Hound)
- Torsion may be more common in dogs with pleural effusion
- Right-middle and left-cranial lung lobes most commonly affected

DIAGNOSIS

Radiography
- Consolidated lung lobe

- Lung lobe edges visible
- Bronchus in an atypical direction (suspect torsion)
- Torsion may be obscured by secondary pleural effusion
  - Transudate
  - Haemorrhage
  - Chyle

Bronchoscopy
Visualisation of twisted bronchus.

CLINICAL FEATURES

- Dyspnoea that gets progressively worse
- Cough
- Lethargy, dullness, pyrexia, anorexia
- Muffled respiratory and cardiac sounds

THERAPY

- Treat the underlying cause as soon as possible to reduce the chances of irreversible collapse
- Lobectomy if irreversible lung change or if there is torsion

- Single, forced, lung inflation to reverse anaesthesia-induced atelectasis
- Attend to the pleural effusion if significant before surgical exploration

---

Note: This is a list of respiratory diseases that are recognised to occur in dogs and cats but are relatively rare or difficult to define accurately, and have not been discussed in any detail in this book. Inflammatory Laryngitis, Granulomatous Laryngitis, Laryngeal Neoplasia, Tracheal Neoplasia, Bronchial Neoplasia, Broncho-oesophageal Fistula, Bronchopulmonary Dysplasia, Primary Ciliary Dyskinesia, Lipid Pneumonia, Pulmonary Metastatic Calcification and Pulmonary Toxins. In addition to this list, the following conditions, which are described in this book, could be viewed as reasonably rare or difficult to define and diagnose: Bronchiectasis, Pulmonary Contusion, Lung Lobe Torsion, Emphysema, Lung Cavitary Lesions, Acute Respiratory Distress Syndrome.

19 DISEASES OF THE PLEURA AND MEDIASTINUM

Diseases of the pleural space typically result in varying degrees of pleural effusion. This is the most important consideration regarding pleural disease in cats and dogs.

PLEURAL EFFUSIONS

A small quantity of serous fluid is normally present in the pleural space but is not detectable on radiography. The identification of even minimal increases in pleural fluid is abnormal. However, the importance of pleural effusion is often related to the volume and its effect on respiratory function.

EFFUSION TYPES

Pleural (and ascitic fluid) should routinely be tapped to determine the type of effusion and its classification. Once this has been done, the diagnostic pathway can be decided. Whilst Table 19.1 classifies effusions by a number of categories, simply determining its character (colour and transparency) and specific gravity (SG) is often sufficient to classify it – this can therefore usually be done in-house.

- True transudates
  - Translucent
  - Colourless
  - Serous
  - Low protein, cellularity and specific gravity
- Modified transudates
  - Opaque
  - Coloured yellow to pink
  - Moderate protein, cellularity and specific gravity
  - Most true transudates become 'modified' after a short period
  - Opaque
  - Coloured yellow to brown
  - High protein, cellularity and specific gravity
  - May contain organisms (*pyothorax*)
- Chyle
  - Opaque
  - Milky-white to blood-tinged
  - Moderate protein
  - High cellularity, lipid content (triglycerides) and specific gravity
  - Large numbers of lymphocytes
- Blood (*haemothorax*)
- Air (*pneumothorax*)

AETIOLOGY

Many diseases can result in different types of effusion.

True and modified transudates
- Hypoproteinaemia
  - Protein-losing enteropathies, malabsorption and maldigestion

Table 19.1   The classification of pleural effusions

Effusion Type	Transparency	Colour	Specific Gravity	Protein Content (g/l)	Cell Count per µl	Predominant Cell Type
True Transudate	Translucent Clear	Yellow or colourless	<1.018	<25	<1500 (–)	n/a
Modified Transudate	Partially opaque Turbid	Yellow to pink	>1.018	>30	1500– 5000 (+)	Variable **Note:** A few RBCs are not uncommon (PCV <5%)
Exudate	Opaque Turbid	Yellow to brown	>1.035	>30	>5000 (+++)	Neutrophil
Chyle	Opaque Turbid	White or pink	>1.030	>25	1500– 10 000 (++)	Lymphocyte TGs are very high compared to serum

- ○ Hepatic failure (reduced albumin production)
- ○ Starvation
- ○ Severe intestinal parasitism
- ○ Protein-losing nephropathy
- ○ Amyloidosis
- • Right-sided congestive heart failure in the dog (more typically causes ascites)
- • Left-sided congestive heart failure in the cat
- • Systemic illness
- • Immune-mediated diseases (very rare cause of pleural effusion)
- • Lung-lobe torsion
- • Allergic or anaphylactic reactions
- • Neoplasia
- • Diaphragmatic hernia

Exudates

- • Many of the conditions that cause transudates
- • Active inflammatory processes
- • Bacterial infections
  - ○ Bacteria from bite wounds
  - ○ Migrating foreign bodies
  - ○ Inhaled foreign bodies
- ○ Penetrating wounds of the chest wall
- ○ *Nocardia* and *Actinomyces* spp, mycobacteria
- ○ *Streptococcus*, *Staphylococcus*, *Proteus*, *Pasteurella* spp, *Escherichia coli*
- • Feline infectious peritonitis virus infection (wet form: pyogranulomatous pleuritis)
- • Neoplasia
- • Thoracic trauma
- • Mediastinal disease

Chyle

- • Idiopathic in the majority of cases
- • Thoracic duct rupture (rare, probably unlikely cause)
- • Inflammatory processes
- • Lung lobe torsion
- • Neoplasia
- • Mediastinal disease
- • Mediastinal lymphosarcoma
- • Congestive heart failure (cats)
- • Cardiomyopathy (cats) – very common cause of chylothorax
- • Pericardial disease
- • Heartworm disease

Haemothorax
- Coagulopathies
- Trauma
- Blood-vessel erosion
- Infections, abscessation, neoplasia
- Inflammatory processes

Pneumothorax
- Trauma to the chest wall (open pneumothorax)
- Damage to the airways and lung tissue
- Rupture of bullae (spontaneous pneumothorax)
- Idiopathic
- Iatrogenic

> **Note:** Pleural mesothelioma is seen in dogs, but is very rare and will give clinical signs due to development of pleural effusion.

In *tension pneumothorax*, the air is trapped in the pleural space during expiration, causing lung collapse. *Pneumomediastinum* can be caused by the same mechanisms and can be spontaneous and self-limiting.

CLINICAL FEATURES

Certain features and clinical signs can be attributed to the specific underlying diseases, but fluid or air accumulation compromises lung expansion, so the clinical presentation can be the same irrespective of the underlying cause.
- Varying degrees of respiratory embarrassment
  - Tachypnoea
  - Dyspnoea
  - Orthopnoea
    - Dogs – remain standing, reluctant to lie down
    - Cats – sternal recumbency, abducted elbows
- Exercise intolerance (dogs)

- Cyanosis at rest or after minimal exertion
- Collapse
- Death
- Weight loss (chronic pleural effusion)
  - Chylothorax
  - Neoplasia
- Inappetance, anorexia
- Pyrexia (pyothorax)
- Paraneoplastic signs
- Other signs of congestive heart failure
- Muffled heart and airway sounds
- Altered thoracic resonance on chest percussion
  - Pleural fluid line
  - Increase in chest resonance (pneumothorax)
- Abdominal changes
  - Distension with concurrent ascites
  - Empty if large abdominal organs have herniated

DIAGNOSIS

Radiography (with caution)
- Homogenous, ground-glass appearance
- Pleural fluid lines
- Lung-lobe compression
- Pleural fissure lines
- Visible lung-lobe borders
- Hyperlucency (with pneumothorax)
- Widened mediastinum

Ultrasonography
- Fluid identification
- Mediastinal examination
- Guided biopsy sampling

Echocardiography
Evidence of congestive heart failure and associated cardiac causes.

Thoracocentesis
- Fluid analysis
  - Colour
  - Specific gravity

- ○ Protein and lipid content (triglyceride levels)
- ○ Turbidity
- ○ Cellularity
- ○ Cytology and culture (aerobic, anaerobic and acid-fast staining)
- Surgical exploration

The underlying cause of pleural effusion may not be readily identifiable. In up to 30% of cases it will not be identified. This is a particular problem with chylothorax in dogs.

THERAPEUTIC TECHNIQUES

Thoracocentesis

- For the immediate relief of life-threatening respiratory distress
- Rapid improvement in respiratory function
- Right or left side of the chest
- Pleural catheters if repeated thoracocentesis required
- Continuous or intermittent drainage
- Catheters can be left in place for 10–14 days
- Pleural lavage in cases of pyothorax

Surgery

- Break down adhesions
- Open pockets of effusion
- Allow accurate pleural catheter placement
- Obtain diagnostic samples
- Remove neoplasms
- Repair diaphragmatic hernias
- Identify cause and treat unresolving or recurrent pneumothorax

TREATMENT OF UNDERLYING CAUSE

Note: Not until adequate chest drainage has been accomplished.

Hypoproteinaemia

- Treat the gastrointestinal, renal or hepatic causes
- Feed a protein diet of high biological value and high bioavailability
- Anti-inflammatory agents for most gastrointestinal causes
- Glucocorticosteroids, immunosuppressive and cytotoxic agents
- Vitamins, minerals etc. for hepatic support
- Improve glomerular function (e.g. angiotensin-converting enzyme inhibitors)

Congestive heart failure

(see Chapter 6)

Haemothorax

- Thoracocentesis sufficient to alleviate dyspnoea
- Whole blood transfusions
- Vitamin K_1 supplementation (rodenticide poisoning)
- Immunosuppressive agents for immune-mediated causes of haemorrhage

Pyothorax

- Must be treated vigorously
- Thoracocentesis, through placed thoracostomy tubes, until only small quantities of sterile serous fluid are obtained (50 ml/day/dog)
- Usually requires 7–10 days of drainage
- Pleural lavage 2–4 times daily (20 ml/kg body weight)
- Antibacterial agents
  - ○ Culture and sensitivity testing
  - ○ Delay in obtaining results
    - – Empirically: Ampicillin at 40 mg/kg q8h + metronidazole at 30 mg/kg q12h
  - ○ Can be difficult to grow some organisms, e.g. *Nocardia* spp
  - ○ Synthetic penicillins (β-lactam agents, penicillin G, cephalosporins)
  - ○ Macrolides and lincosamides (e.g. clindamycin)

- ○ Potentiated sulphonamides (might be inactivated by pus)
- Treatment for at least six weeks (four months in the case of nocardiosis) at very high doses is imperative
- Surgical exploration and resection of devitalised tissues in chronic, poorly responsive pyothorax, is advised

Chylothorax

- Initial thoracocentesis
- Monitor for hyponatraemia and hypokalaemia
- Treatment of congestive heart failure (mainly cats)
- Dietary control
  - ○ Restrict dietary fat intake (commercial products preferred)
  - ○ Feed a high protein, high carbohydrate diet with vitamin supplementation
  - ○ Medium-chain triglyceride dietary fats

- Surgical ligation of thoracic duct +/– pericardiectomy if:
  - ○ Dietary management is unsuccessful
  - ○ There is a chronic build up of chyle in the thorax
- Diuresis to minimise volume of fluid
- Rutin supplementation is of questionable value

PROGNOSIS

Prognosis depends on the nature of the effusion and its cause. Pleural effusion is a serious condition and may require radical and often long-term therapy. In many situations the condition will not be resolved. Prognosis is grave with neoplastic causes, while pyothorax is usually curable with the proper intervention. Unresolvable chylous effusions will result in debility and cachexia in the long term, while most cases of pneumothorax resolve spontaneously.

DISEASES OF THE MEDIASTINUM

Mediastinal disease typically results in mediastinal widening, but mediastinal narrowing can also occur.

AETIOLOGY

- Mediastinitis
  - ○ Foreign body penetration of the oesophagus
  - ○ Abscesses
  - ○ Granulomas
- Oedema
- Haemorrhage
  - ○ Trauma
  - ○ Coagulopathies
  - ○ Neoplasia

- Mediastinal neoplasia
  - ○ Malignant lymphoma – most are T-cell lymphomas
  - ○ Lymphosarcoma
  - ○ Thymic lymphosarcoma in cats
  - ○ Chemodectomas (heart-based, aortic body tumours)
- Lymphadenopathy
  - ○ Inflammatory reaction
  - ○ Neoplasia
  - ○ Infection
- Widening of the caudal mediastinum
  - ○ Congenital pericardiodiaphragmatic hernia
  - ○ Gastro-oesophageal reflux of the stomach through a hiatal hernia
  - ○ Megaoesophagus

Note: *Pneumomediastinum* refers to air in the mediastinal space. Mediastinal structures will be visible on radiography (outer edges of the tracheal wall, the azygous vein, major vessels). It is caused by air escaping from the trachea, bronchi or oesophagus due to trauma, neoplastic erosion, complications of surgery or other investigations, or it may be idiopathic. Air may enter through the thoracic inlet or from the abdomen. Pneumomediastinum should be left to resolve spontaneously, but this can take up to three weeks. Surgical intervention is only required if there is severe, life-threatening dyspnoea.

CLINICAL SIGNS OF MEDIASTINAL DISEASE

Clinical signs of mediastinal disease are referrable to compression of structures.
• Trachea
  ○ Dyspnoea
  ○ Coughing
  ○ Respiratory noise
• Recurrent laryngeal nerve
  ○ Laryngeal paralysis
• Oesophagus
  ○ Dysphagia
  ○ Regurgitation
  ○ Retching
• Vagosympathetic trunk
  ○ Horner's syndrome (miosis, ptosis, third eyelid prolapse and enophthalmos)
• Head and forelimb oedema (vena cava syndrome)
• Signs of right-sided cardiac failure (pericardiodiaphragmatic hernia)

DIAGNOSIS

Radiography
• Mediastinal widening
• Displacement of cranial lung lobes
• Soft tissue density cranial mediastinal area
• Cardiomegaly
• Megaoesophagus

Ultrasonography
• Distinguish soft tissue from free fluid
• Assists guided sampling

Surgical exploration
• Confirm mediastinal involvement
• Obtain diagnostic samples

DISEASES OF THE DIAPHRAGM AND CHEST WALL

Most of these problems have been discussed elsewhere in this book. Conditions to consider include:
• Diaphragmatic hernia
  ○ Congenital forms
  ○ Acquired forms
• Flail-chest segments and rib fractures

• *Pectus excavatum*
  ○ Congenital chondrosternal depression (funnel chest)
  ○ Rare condition
  ○ Signs of respiratory compromise
  ○ Diagnosis
    – Physical palpation
    – Thoracic radiography
  ○ Treatment is by surgical correction

SECTION 4
CARDIOPULMONARY RESUSCITATION

20 CARDIOPULMONARY RESUSCITATION

Cardiopulmonary resuscitation (CPR) is the action taken to restore ventilation and circulation to vital tissues (See also inside back cover).

- *Cerebrocardiovascular resuscitation* is a newer term, which emphasises the importance of preserving cerebral function.
- The survival rate for CPR in a dog or cat, following true cardiopulmonary arrest (CPA), is poor, with a range of 5–20%.
- CPR is not usually performed on animals in which death is associated with end-stage disease, death is expected or CPR is unlikely to be successful.
- CPR is usually performed when cardiopulmonary arrest is unexpected and the life-threatening process leading to the arrest is considered to be reversible.

CARDIOPULMONARY ARREST (CPA)

- Cessation of ventilation and circulation
- CPA may occur acutely, usually due to a single devastating factor, or chronically, with a multifactorial cause

CLINICAL FEATURES OF CPA

- Apnoea
- Absence of a palpable pulse, palpable apex beat or heart sounds
- Central eye position
- Pupils fixed and dilated (in 30–45 seconds)
- Cornea becomes dry
- Mucous membranes – dirty grey colour (or cyanosis or pallor)
- Absence of cranial nerve reflexes
- Muscle hypotonicity
- Agonal gasping – poor prognostic indicator
- ECG may show ventricular fibrillation, sinus bradycardia or asystole
- ECG will appear normal, with electromechanical dissociation (EMD)

EQUIPMENT AND FACILITIES FOR CPR

- Endotracheal tubes
- Airway suctioning
- Laryngoscope
- Tracheostomy tubes
- ECG monitoring
- Pulse oximetry
- Capnography
- Electrical defibrillator
- Fluids and administration sets
- Intravenous catheters, syringes and needles
- Large-gauge and long intravenous catheters for catheterisation of the jugular vein
- Water manometer set for measurement of central venous pressure (CVP)
- Emergency drugs and clearly-displayed dosage chart
- Instruments for a rapid thoracotomy and pericardiectomy

DR ABC

The mnemonic Dr ABCDEF can be helpful for remembering the steps of CPR during a crisis.

- D – Danger
- R – Responsiveness
- A – Airway
- B – Breathing
- C – Circulation
- D – Drugs
- E – Electrical defibrillation
- F – Follow up

D – DANGER

Assess the danger, to yourself and others, of handling an animal. Will it bite or scratch?

R – RESPONSE

Is the patient responsive? What's the level of consciousness?

A – AIRWAY

- Intubation is the best means to ensure an airway and deliver oxygen
- Check endotracheal tube is not occluded (particularly toy breeds and cats) with mucus, blood or debris

B – BREATHING

- Positive pressure ventilation with 100% oxygen (manual or mechanical)
- Ventilate at 25–30 breaths per minute
- Inflation should provide significant (supranormal) chest-wall expansion, but it is also important to allow the lungs to deflate fully after each ventilation

> **Note:** Respiratory arrest or apnoea is not uncommon with an anaesthetic overdose. If there is a good heart beat and pulse, positive pressure ventilation is usually all that is required until the anaesthetic drugs are distributed or metabolised and their effects dissipate.

C – CIRCULATION

External cardiac compression

Blood flow is achieved by one of two mechanisms, depending upon the size of animal and chest-wall compliance.

Cardiac pump
- Cardiac massage – squeezes the ventricles and great vessels by compressing the ribs over the cardiac area
- Relies on chest-wall compliance (i.e. the ribs are compressible over the cardiac area), therefore only effective in cats, puppies, very narrow-chested dogs (e.g. Greyhound) and dogs no heavier than 20 kg

Thoracic pump
- Compression of the chest wall (at its widest point) causes an increase in intrathoracic pressure, thus compressing the great vessels, to produce forward flow (backward flow is prevented by venous and cardiac valves)
- On chest decompression, venous blood is then drawn into the vacuum, providing venous return to the heart
- Synchronous lung inflation and chest wall compression maximises intrathoracic pressure
- A compression rate of 60–120 per minute (depending on breed) is sustained

SECTION 4

- It is important that the endotracheal tube is *proximal to the thoracic inlet* when implementing the thoracic pump mechanism
- Chest compression should be abrupt and allow sufficient decompression time for venous return

Abdominal binding

Bandage hind legs and abdomen. This increases venous return and restricts diaphragmatic movement facilitating the generation of higher intrathoracic pressure. It also discourages blood flow to the abdomen thus increasing cerebral flow.

Internal cardiac compression

Indications
- Dogs greater than 20 kg
- Dogs that are broad chested with poor chest-wall compressibility
- Pneumothorax
- Pericardial tamponade
- Flail chest
- Diaphragmatic hernia
- Hypovolaemia
- Obesity

Technique
- Requires rapid (but careful) thoracotomy (full length) and retraction with rib retractors
- The pericardium is opened

Tip: To open the pericardium quickly, hook a finger around the cardio-diaphragmatic ligament (found at the cardiac apex) and lift it so that it can be cut with a pair of scissors. It is important not to lift the heart excessively as this may distort the great vessels and occlude flow.

- Massage ('milk') heart gently from apex to base
- Rate dictated by ventricular filling – approximately 80–120/min
- The heart must be kept warm and moist, which can be achieved by pouring warm fluids into the thorax
- Cross-clamping of the descending aorta (for up to 35 minutes) with atraumatic forceps improves cerebral and coronary blood flow

Advantages of internal cardiac compression
- Two to three times more effective than external cardiac compression
  - Internal cardiac compression provides 50–70% of cardiac output
  - External cardiac compression provides 10–20% of cardiac output
- Accurate intraventricular injections can be made
- Adequacy of venous return can be visualised
- Lung inflation can be assessed
- Certain arrhythmias can be seen and diagnosed (e.g. ventricular fibrillation, asystole)

Disadvantages of internal cardiac compression
- Time to perform a thoracotomy delays continued cardiac compression
- Difficult to perform
- Unfamiliarity with direct cardiac massage may reduce effectiveness
- If resuscitation is successful, post-operative sepsis may pose a problem subsequently

D – DRUGS

The choice of drugs is dependent upon the situation and requires an ECG facility.

CARDIOPULMONARY RESUSCITATION

TABLE 20.1 Routes for drug administration during CPR, in order of preference

Route of Administration	Technique	Comments
Central Vein	Catheterisation with a long catheter so that the tip is within the cranial vena cava	• Injection of drugs • Rapid fluid administration • Monitoring central venous pressure
Pulmonary Vein	During open chest CPR – use small-gauge needle	• Drugs reach the heart effectively
Intratracheal (I/T)	Pass a long catheter through the endotracheal tube to the bifurcation of the trachea	• Double the i/v doses + saline (0.5 ml/kg) • Useful for atropine, adrenaline and lidocaine
Intracardiac Injections	Injection of drugs directly into the ventricles	• Hazardous
Peripheral Veins (I/V)	Preplaced cephalic or saphenous vein catheter	• Drugs take excessive length of time to reach the heart, if they reach it at all

TABLE 20.2 Treatment of arrhythmias during CPR

ECG Rhythm	Description	Treatment
Asystole	Heart stopped • No heart sounds • No pulse • No visible heart movement • 'Flat-line' on ECG	• Warm heart – raise body temperature • Atropine • Methoxamine • Fluid loading • Maintaining CPR • Adrenaline
Electromechanical Dissociation (EMD)	ECG appears normal, but no cardiac contractions or movement.	• Steroids • Methoxamine • Calcium • Adrenaline • Bicarbonate • Maintain CPR
Ventricular Fibrillation	• Irregular and uncoordinated contractions of ventricles • Irregular deflections on ECG • Feels like a 'can of wriggling worms'	• Convert fine ventricular fibrillation to coarse fibrillation with adrenaline • Electrical defibrillation
Sinus Bradycardia	Normal ECG and cardiac contraction with a pulse, but at a slow rate	• Atropine • Dobutamine or dopamine • Restore normal temperature • Correct hypokalaemia
Idioventricular Rhythm	• ECG – ventricular escapes at a slow rate • Very weak or absent pulse	• Poor prognosis

TABLE 20.3 Doses of emergency drugs

Drug	Route	Dose Rate	Dose
Adrenaline (1:1000) (1 mg/ml)	i/v	0.2 mg/kg	2 ml per 10 kg
Adrenaline (1:10000) (0.1 mg/ml)	i/v	0.2 mg/kg	20 ml per 10 kg
Atropine (600 µg/ml)	i/v	40 µg/kg	0.7 ml per 10 kg
Bicarbonate 8.4% (1 mEq/ml)	i/v	1 mmol/kg (1 mEq/kg)	10 ml per 10 kg
Lidocaine 2% (20 mg/ml)	i/v	2 mg/kg; repeat 3–4 times ($^1/_4$ to $^1/_2$ dose for cats)	1 ml per 10 kg per bolus
Electrical	External	4 J/kg	10–50 Joules per 10 kg
Defibrillation (Joules = watt seconds)	Internal	0.1–0.5 J/kg	1–5 Joules per 10 kg

E – ELECTRICAL DEFIBRILLATION

- Used for the conversion of ventricular fibrillation to sinus rhythm.
- Electrical (direct current (DC)) defibrillation temporarily interrupts ventricular fibrillation thus allowing the intrinsic pacemaker (sinus node) to resume its normal rhythm. Chemical defibrillation is ineffective in small animals.

External defibrillation

- Conducting gel is applied to the paddles and the chest wall over the cardiac area
- The paddles are then placed over the left and right sides of the cardiac apex
- The operator and all staff must be insulated from the animal and paddles before DC shock is given
- If no response is seen on ECG then cardiac massage is resumed, the defibrillator turned to the next power setting and the procedure repeated

Internal defibrillation

The internal paddles are covered in saline-soaked swabs and placed opposite each other, in contact with the heart. The procedure is carried out as described above.

F – FOLLOW-UP

If CPR is successful in resuming normal cardiac function, continued support is required.

- Fluids should be continued at 5 ml/kg/hour until recovery
- Dopamine or dobutamine infusion helps to maintain cardiac output and improve renal bloodflow
- Minimise cerebral oedema and intra-cranial pressure
  - Raise head position
  - Steroids at high doses – Solu-Medrone (methylprednisolone) at 30 mg/kg slow i/v
  - Furosemide at 4 mg/kg
  - Hyperventilation to avoid hypercapnia and hypoxia
  - Diazepam to control seizures (0.5 mg/kg slow i/v to effect)
- Bladder should be catheterised, emptied and urine output monitored
  - Optimal urine output is 1–1.5 ml/kg/hour

CARDIOPULMONARY RESUSCITATION

- o If less than this, increase fluid administration, dopamine infusion and furosemide
- Body temperature (measured by an oesophageal probe rather than a rectal thermometer)
  - o Should be at least 33.3°C prior to closure of a thoracotomy
  - o Irrigation of the chest (after open cardiac massage) with warmed (38°C) fluids assists in restoring body temperature
  - o Increase room temperature
  - o Rectal lavage with warm water
- Closure of the thoracotomy will involve clipping and cleaning the incision wound
- Analgesia should be provided, e.g. by intercostal nerve blocks with long-acting local anaesthetics (e.g. bupivacaine).
- Intravenous antibiotic should be administered

- Positive pressure ventilation is continued until spontaneous breathing resumes
- Endotracheal tube and trachea should be cleared of any discharge or debris
- Oxygen by nasal catheter (or oxygen-enriched cage)
- Intensive nursing following successful CPR is essential

PROGNOSIS

Prognosis is very poor and CPR is frequently unsuccessful. It is also time consuming, and, if carried out properly, is very expensive. The prognosis improves if there is immediate availability of at least three trained (and practised) personnel and if the time delay between CPA, its recognition and the institution of CPR is short. Despite successful CPR, prolonged CPA can result in serious neurological deficits, such as blindness, coma or seizures.

SECTION 5
APPENDICES

APPENDIX 1

COMMON BREED PREDISPOSITIONS TO CARDIORESPIRATORY DISEASE IN DOGS

Listed below are some common breed predispositions to cardiorespiratory disease in dogs. This is not an exhaustive list, but aims to offer the clinician some guidelines on what to consider when formulating a differential diagostic list. The breed prevalence may vary between countries or even regions within countries.

ABBREVIATIONS

CARDIAC DISEASES

- AVVD – AV valve dysplasia
- DCM – Dilated cardiomyopathy
- PAS – Persistent atrial standstill
- PDA – Patent ductus arteriosus
- PE – Pericardial effusion
- PS – Pulmonic stenosis
- SAS – Subaortic stenosis
- SSS – Sick sinus syndrome
- ToF – Tetralogy of Fallot
- MVD – Mitral valve disease
- VSD – Ventricular septal defect

RESPIRATORY DISEASES

- BUAS – Brachycephalic upper airway syndrome
- CD – Ciliary dyskinesia
- HT – Hypoplastic trachea
- LP – Laryngeal paralysis
- IPF – Idiopathic pulmonary fibrosis
- TC – Tracheal collapse

APPENDIX TABLE 1.1   Breed predispositions to cardiorespiratory disease

Breed	Cardiac	Respiratory
Beagle	PS	
Bichon Frise		CD
Border Collie	PDA, VSD	
Boston Terrier	MVD, VSD	
Boxer	SAS, PS, DCM, PE	
Cavalier King Charles Spaniel	MVD, PDA, PAS, PS	BUAS
Cairn Terrier	SSS	IPF
Chihuahua	PS, MVD	
Chow Chow	PS	
Cocker Spaniel	DCM, MVD, PDA, PS	
Dobermann	DCM	
English Bulldog	SAS, PS, ToF, VSD	HT, BUAS
English Bull Terrier	AVVD, SAS	
English Springer Spaniel	PAS	
Fox Terrier	PS, MVD	
German Shepherd Dog	PDA, SAS, DCM, PE, AVVD	
Golden Retriever	DCM, SAS, PE	
Gordon Setter	MVD, DCM	CD
Great Dane	AVVD, DCM, PE	
Irish Setter	MVD, DCM, PDA	LP
Irish Wolfhound	DCM	
Keeshound	ToF, VSD	
Labrador	DCM, PS, AVVD	LP
Mastiff	PS	
Miniature Poodle	PDA, MVD	TC
Miniature Schnauzer	SSS, MVD, PS	
Newfoundland	SAS, DCM	
Old English Sheepdog	DCM, AVVD, PAS	
Pekinese	MVD	BUAS
Pomeranian	PDA	
Pug		BUAS
Rottweiller	SAS	
Samoyed	SAS, PS	
St Bernard	DCM, PE	
Schnauzer	MVD, PS	
Shih Tzu	PS	
Shetland Sheepdog	PDA	
Springer Spaniel	DCM, PAS, VSD	CD
West Highland White Terrier	PS, SSS, VSD	IPF
Yorkshire Terrier	MVD, PS	TC

APPENDIX 2

CALCULATING CONSTANT RATE INFUSIONS OF LIGNOCAINE AND DOBUTAMINE

Delivery rate (ml/hr) of the infusion

$$= \frac{\text{dose rate of drug (µg/kg/min)} \times \text{body weight (kg)} \times \text{volume of fluid in bag (ml)} \times 60}{\text{quantity of drug (ml) added to fluids} \times 1000}$$

APPENDIX TABLE 2.1 Calculation of constant rate infusion for *lidocaine* [replace 25 ml of 500 ml bag of fluids with 25 ml of 2% lidocaine without adrenaline (20 mg/ml)]

Body Weight (kg)		10	20	30	40	50
Dose Rate	**Fluid Rate**					
(µg/kg/min)	**(ml/h)**					
25		15	30	45	60	75
50		30	60	90	120	150
70		45	90	135	180	225

APPENDIX TABLE 2.2 Calculation of constant rate infusion for *dobutamine* [replace 20 ml of 500 ml bag of fluids with 20 ml of dobutamine (12.5 mg/ml)]

Body Weight (kg)		10	20	30	40	50
Dose Rate	**Fluid Rate**					
(µg/kg/min)	**(ml/h)**					
5		6	12	18	24	30
7.5		9	18	27	36	45
10		12	24	36	48	60

APPENDIX 3
DIGOXIN USE IN THE DOG

(See pp. 68 and 77)

Causes of a persistently high heart rate in dogs receiving digoxin for atrial fibrillation

- Elevation of the heart rate in-clinic due to nervousness at the time of examination – may require 24-hour Holter to determine average heart rate at home
- Inadequate control of the congestive failure signs – sympathetic drive is still high
- Dehydration/hypotension due to over-diuresis/-vasodilation
- Inadequate serum levels of digoxin
- Concurrent medical disease, e.g. renal failure
- Advanced myocardial failure and end-stage heart disease
- Heart rate poorly responsive to digoxin – needs additional antiarrhythmic drugs

APPENDIX TABLE 3.1 Digoxin starting dose in dogs

Body Weight (kg)	Tablet Strength (μg)	Tablet Dose (q12h)
1–5	62.5 (PG)	$^1/_2$
6–13	62.5 (PG)	1
14–23	125	1
24–36	125	$1^1/_2$
>37	250	1

Note: Dobermann dose is one 125 μg tablet q12h.

APPENDIX 4

SOME NORMAL ECHOCARDIOGRAPHIC VALUES FOR DOGS AND CATS

APPENDIX TABLE 4.1   Normal left ventricular (LV), left atrial (LA) and aortic (Ao) diameter values for **cats** (Bonagura *et al.* 1985)

Parameter	Measurement (mm)
LVd	11.0–16.0
LVs	6.0–10.0
IVSd	2.5–5.0
IVSs	5.0–9.0
LVPWd	2.5–5.0
LVPWs	4.0–9.0
LA	8.5–12.5
Ao	6.5–11.0
FS%	29–55%

APPENDIX TABLE 4.2   Normal left atrial diameter for **dogs** obtained by 2-D measurement (long axis and short axis) as described by Rishniw (2000)

Weight (kg)	Left Atrium Long Axis Diameter Range (mm)	Left Atrium Short Axis Diameter Range (mm)
5	16–27	10–23
10	21–32	14–26
15	25–36	17–29
20	29–40	20–32
30	35–45	25–37
40	38–48	28–42
50	38–50	29–43
Ratio to aorta	<2:1	<1.6:1

APPENDICES

APPENDIX TABLE 4.3   Published normal left ventricular internal diameter measurements and fractional shortening for individual breeds of dog

Breed	Parameter	LVDd (mm)	LVDs (mm)	FS (%)	Reference
Irish Wolfhound	Mean (SD)	53.2 (4.0)	35.4 (2.8)	34 (4.5)	Vollmar (1999a)
Irish Wolfhound	Mean (SD)				Brownlie & Cobb
	Male	53.3 (4.5)	38.6 (3.7)	28.2 (4.3)	(1999)
	Female	51.8 (4.0)	36.9 (4.2)	29.1 (4.3)	
Spanish Mastiff	Mean (SD)	47 (1.4)	29 (1.1)	39 (1.6)	Bayon *et al.* (1994)
Great Dane	Range	44–59	34–45	18–36	Koch *et al.* (1996)
Deerhound	Mean (SD)	51 (5)	34 (5)	33 (6)	Vollmar (1998)
Newfoundland	Mean (SD)	45.3 (3.8)	33.7 (2.9)	25 (2.9)	Dukes-McEwan (1999)
Saluki	Mean (SD)	45 (4)	33 (4)	28	Brownlie (1999)
Greyhound	Range	40–49	29–38	17–35	Page *et al.* (1993)
English Pointer	Mean (SD)	39.2 (2.4)	25.3 (2.4)	35.5 (4.0)	Sisson & Schaeffer (1991)
Golden Retriever	Range	37–51	18–35	27–55	Morrison *et al.* (1992)
Dobermann	Normal range	32.7–45.2	25.7–37.9	13–30	O'Grady & Horne (1995)
Afghan	Range	33–52	20–37	24–48	Morrison *et al.* (1992)
Boxer	Range	40 (4.5)	27 (4.0)	32 (7)	Herrtage (1994)
Cocker Spaniel	Mean (SD)	33.8 (3.3)	22.2 (2.8)	34.3 (4.5)	Gooding *et al.* (1986)
Corgi	Range	28–40	12–23	33–57	Morrison *et al.* (1992)
Cavalier King Charles Spaniel	Mean (SD)	29 (3)	20 (2.5)	33 (4.5)	Häggström (2000)
Beagle	Range	18–33	8–27	20–70	Crippa (1992)
Miniature Poodle	Range	16–28	8–16	35–57	Morrison *et al.* (1992)

SECTION 5

APPENDIX 5

NORMAL ECG VALUES FOR DOGS AND CATS

APPENDIX TABLE 5.1   Normal ECG values for dogs and cats (Tilley 1992)

Parameter	Canine	Normal Value	Feline	Normal Value
Rate	Adult	70–160	Adult	120–240
	Giant breeds	60–140	Average rate	190–200
	Toy breeds	70–180		
	Puppy	70–220		
P Wave Duration	Maximum	0.04 sec	Maximum	0.04 sec
	Giant breeds maximum	0.05 sec		
P Wave Amplitude	Maximum	0.4 mV	Maximum	0.2 mV
P-R Interval	Range	0.06–0.13 sec	Range	0.05–0.09 sec
QRS Duration	Maximum	0.05 sec	Maximum	0.04 sec
	Large breeds maximum	0.06 sec		
R Wave Amplitude	Maximum	2.5 mV	Maximum	0.9 mV
	Large breeds maximum	2.0 mV		
S-T segment	Maximum depression	0.2 mV	No depression	n/a
	Maximum elevation	0.15 mV	No elevation	
T Wave	Can be positive, negative or biphasic	$<^1/_4$ of R wave amplitude	Can be positive, negative or biphasic	
			Maximum	0.3 mV
Q-T Interval	Range at normal heart rate	0.15–0.25 sec	Range at normal heart rate	0.12–0.18 sec
Mean Electrical Axis	Range	+40° to +100°	Range	0 to +160°

Note: Some measurements differ for deep-chested dogs less than two years of age.

APPENDIX 6

CLASSIFICATION OF PLEURAL EFFUSIONS

Pleural and ascitic fluid should routinely be tapped to determine the type of effusion and its classification. Once this has been done, the diagnostic pathway can be decided. Whilst this table classifies effusion by a number of categories, simply determining its character (colour and transparency) and the SG is often sufficient to classify it – this can usually be done in-house.

APPENDIX TABLE 6.1   The classification of pleural effusions

Effusion Type	Transparency	Colour	Specific Gravity	Protein Content (g/l)	Cell Count per µl	Predominant Cell Type
True Transudate	Translucent Clear	Yellow or colourless	<1.018	<25	<1500	–
Modified Transudate	Partially opaque Turbid	Yellow to pink	>1.018	>30	1500 to 5000	Variable Cell Type Note: A few red cells are not uncommon (PCV <5%)
Exudate	Opaque Turbid	Yellow to brown	>1.035	>30	>5000	Neutrophil
Chyle	Opaque Turbid	White or pink	>1.030	>25	1500 to 10000	Lymphocyte TGs are very high compared to serum

APPENDIX 7

SEDATION REGIMES FOR DOGS AND CATS WITH CARDIORESPIRATORY DISEASE

DOGS

- Suggested sedation regimes for thoracic radiography are those used by the authors
- For effective sedation, dogs must be left undisturbed and given sufficient time for the drug(s) to take effect

Caution: Doses of ACP should be *reduced by ¹/₄–¹/₂* for dogs in congestive failure or dogs that are debilitated.

Caution: Due to their vagal sensitivity, a low dose of ACP must be used in *Boxers* (i.e. one third of standard dose), and the vagal effects of ACP counteracted by combining with pentazocine (at the dose above) given i/m only.

APPENDICES

APPENDIX TABLE 7.1   Dose of acepromazine maleate (ACP 2 mg/ ml)

Route	Dose Rate	Dose
i/m	0.05 mg/kg	0.25 ml per 10 kg (maximum 1 ml for dogs >40 kg)
i/v	0.02 mg/kg	0.1 ml per 10 kg (maximum 0.4 ml for dogs >40 kg)

APPENDIX TABLE 7.2   Drug to be combined with ACP

Sedative Drug	Route	Dose Rate	Dose
Butorphanol	i/m or i/v	0.1–0.2 mg/kg	0.1–0.2 ml per 10 kg
Buprenorphine	i/m or i/v	0.01 mg/kg	0.33 ml per 10 kg
Pentazocine	i/m	2 mg/kg	0.66 ml/10 kg i/m
Pethidine	i/m	2–3 mg/kg	0.4–0.6 ml per 10 kg

Drug concentrations: Butorphanol – Torbugesic 10 mg/ml; Buprenorphine – Vetergesic 0.3 mg/ml; Pentazocine – Fortral 30 mg/ml; Pethidine – 50 mg/ml

CATS

- Suggested sedation regimes for thoracic radiography are those used by the authors
- For effective sedation, cats must be left undisturbed and given sufficient time for the drug(s) to take effect

Caution: Doses should be reduced in cats that are in congestive failure or those that are debilitated.

APPENDIX TABLE 7.3   Sedation regimes for cats with cardiorespiratory disease

Sedative Drug	Route	Dose Rate (mg/kg)	Dose (ml/4 kg)
Midazolam +	Combined i/m	0.25	0.25
Ketamine		+ 5–10	+ 0.2–0.4
Midazolam +	Combined i/v	0.25	0.25
Ketamine		+ 2.5	+ 0.1
Acepromazine	All combined i/m	0.03	0.06
maleate +		+ 0.25	+ 0.25
Midazolam +		+ 10	+ 0.4
Ketamine			
Acepromazine	Combined either	0.05	0.1
maleate +	i/m or i/v	+ 0.3	+ 0.12
Butorphanol			

Drug concentrations: Acepromazine maleate – ACP 2 mg/ml; Butorphanol – Torbugesic 10 mg/ml; Midazolam – Hypnovel 5 mg/ml; Ketamine – Vetalar, Ketaset 100 mg/ml; Propofol – Rapinovet, Propoflo 10 mg/ml

APPENDIX TABLE 7.4   For additional sedation to that used in Appendix Table 7.3, add one of the following

Sedative Drug	Route	Dose Rate (mg/kg)	Dose (ml/4 kg)
Ketamine	i/m	5–10	0.2–0.4
Ketamine	i/v	2.5	0.1
Propofol	i/v slowly	3	1.2

Drug concentrations: Ketamine – Vetalar, Ketaset 100 mg/ml; Propofol – Rapinovet, Propoflo 10 mg/ml

APPENDIX 8

DOSES OF EMERGENCY DRUGS

APPENDIX TABLE 8.1 Doses of emergency drugs

Drug	Route	Dose Rate	Dose
Adrenaline (1:1000) (1 mg/ml)	i/v	0.2 mg/kg	2 ml per 10 kg
Adrenaline (1:10 000) (0.1 mg/ml)	i/v	0.2 mg/kg	20 ml per 10 kg
Atropine (600 µg/ml)	i/v	40 µg/kg	0.7 ml per 10 kg
Bicarbonate 8.4% (1 mEq/ml)	i/v	1 mmol/kg (1 mEq/kg)	10 ml per 10 kg
Lidocaine 2% (21 mg/ml)	i/v	2 mg/kg repeat 3–4 times ($^1/_4$–$^1/_2$ dose for cats)	1 ml per 10 kg per bolus
Electrical Defibrillation (Joules = watt-second)	External	4 J/kg	10–50 Joules per 10 kg
	Internal	0.1–0.5 J/kg	1–5 Joules per 10 kg

DRUG GLOSSARY

Listed below, in alphabetical order, are some of the drugs commonly used in cardiology and respiratory medicine, and their recommended dosages. For more detail regarding the use of these agents, consult other sections of this book.

The recommended doses are derived from various sources, including the authors' own experience, standard veterinary textbooks, formularies and data sheets for licensed veterinary products. For detailed information regarding uses, contraindications and side effects the reader should consult appropriate formularies and the product data sheets.

See Appendices for:
- Constant rate infusion tables for lidocaine and dobutamine (Appendix 2)
- Digoxin starting dose (Appendix 3)
- Sedation regimes and doses for cats and dogs with cardiorespiratory disease (Appendix 7)
- Emergency drugs (Appendix 8)

DRUG GLOSSARY TABLE   Commonly used drugs and their dosages

Drug	Species	Dose
Aminophylline	Dog	10 mg/kg q8–12h po
	Cat	5 mg/kg q12h po or slow i/v (diluted)
Amiodarone	Dog	10–15 mg/kg q12h po for 5–10 days, reducing to 5–10 mg/kg q24h (to minimum effective dose)
Amlodipine	Cat	0.625–1.25 mg per cat q24h (to q12h) (start at lowest dose)
	Dog	0.05–0.1 mg/kg q12–24h (start at lowest dose)
Aspirin	Dog	5 mg/kg daily
(Anti-platelet-aggregation dose)	Cat	5–30 mg/cat twice a week
Atenolol	Dog	0.25–2.0 mg/kg q12h po (start at lowest dose)
	Cat	1–2 mg/kg q12–24h po (start at lowest dose)
Atropine	Dog/cat	40 μg/kg s/c or i/v
Benazepril	Dog	0.25 mg/kg q24h po (increase to q12h in advanced cases)
	Cat	0.5 mg/kg q12–24h po
Bromhexine	Dog	2 mg/kg q12h po
	Cat	1 mg/kg q24h po

DRUG GLOSSARY TABLE   (*continued*)

Drug	Species	Dose
Butorphanol	Dog	0.5–1.0 mg/kg i/m, s/c or q6–12h po
(Antitussive dose)	Cat	0.1 mg/kg i/m
Clenbuterol	Dog	1–5 µg/kg q8–12h
	Cat	1 µg/kg q12–24h
Co-amilozide	Dog/cat	1–3 mg/kg q12h (usually used concurrently
(Amiloride +		with furosemide)
hydrochlorothiazide)		
Codeine	Dog	0.5–2 mg/kg q8–12/h po
Cyproheptadine	Dog/Cat	0.1–0.5 mg/kg q8–12h po
(Serotonin antagonist)		
Dalteparin	Dog/cat	100–200 iu/kg s/c q12h
(Low-molecular-		
weight heparin)		
Dexamethasone	Dog/cat	0.1–0.5 mg/kg i/v, i/m
		5 mg/kg i/v for shock
Dextromethorphan	Dog	0.1–5 mg q8–12h po
Diazepam	Dog/cat	0.1 mg/kg i/v, repeat every few minutes to
(Anti-seizure dose)		a maximum of 0.5 mg/kg
Digoxin	Dog	0.22 mg/m^2 q12 hours (for recommended starting
		dose see Appendix 3, p. 188, also pp. 68 and 77)
	Cat	<4 kg: 0.0625 mg tablet, $^1/_2$ q48h;
		>4 kg: 0.0625 mg tablet, $^1/_2$ q24h
Diltiazem	Dog	1–3 mg/kg q8h po (start at lowest dose)
	Cat	1.6–3.3 mg/kg q8h po; slow release
		(Dilacor XR): 30 mg per cat q24h
Dobutamine	Dog	5.0–10 µg/kg/min i/v (see also
		Appendix Table 2.2, p. 187)
Doxapram	Dog/cat	0.5–1.0 mg/kg i/v
Enalapril	Dog	0.5 mg/kg q24h po (increase to q12h
		in advanced cases)
Enilconazole	Dog/cat	10 mg/kg bid for 14 days
Enoxaparin	Dog/cat	100 iu/kg s/c q12h
(Low-molecular-		
weight heparin)		
Esmolol	Dog/cat	0.05–0.1 mg/kg slow i/v q5min to
		a maximum of 0.5 mg/kg
Etamiphylline	Dog/cat	10–20 mg/kg q8–12h po
Camsylate		14–20 mg/kg q8–12h i/v or s/c

DRUG GLOSSARY TABLE   (continued)

Drug	Species	Dose
Fenbendazole (Treatment of lungworm)	Dog/cat	Mild infection: 100 mg/kg daily for 5–7 days Moderate infection: 50 mg/kg daily for 7–10 days Severe infection: 20 mg/kg daily for 10–14 days
Fish Oils	Dog/cat	Eicosapentaenoeic acid (EPA): 40 mg/kg per day Docosahexanoeic acid (DHA): 25 mg/kg per day
Furosemide (Frusemide)		Starting dose:
	Dog	1–2 mg/kg q12h (up to 4 mg/kg q8h)
	Cat	1 mg/kg q12–24h (up to 2 mg/kg q12h) Acute failure:
	Dog	3–4 mg/kg q2h i/v or i/m
	Cat	1–2 mg/kg q2h i/v or i/m
Glyceryl Trinitrate (2% ointment)	Dog	0.5–5.0 cm topically (depending on size of dog) q6–8h for 3 days
	Cat	0.5 cm q8h topically for 3 days
Heparin	Dog/cat	250 iu/kg q8h
Hydralazine	Dog	Start at 0.5 mg/kg q12h, titrating to a maximum of 2 mg/kg q12h
Hydroxycarbamide (Hydroxyurea) (For polycythaemia)	Dog/cat	50 mg/kg twice a week to start (see Chapter 13, p. 126)
Imidapril	Dog	0.25 mg/kg q24h po (increase to q12h in advanced cases)
Ketoconazole	Dog/cat	5–10 mg/kg q24h
L-carnitine	Dog	50 mg/kg q8h
Lidocaine (Lignocaine)	Dog	2–3 mg/kg slowly i/v every few minutes to a maximum of 9 mg/kg in 20–30 minutes 25–75µg/kg/min i/v infusion (see Appendix Table 2.1, p. 187)
	Cat	0.25–0.75 mg/kg, can repeat after 20 minutes
Magnesium Amino Chelate (200 mg tablets)	Dog	10 mg/kg daily with food
Mexilitine	Dog	5–8 mg/kg q8h po
Morphine	Dog	0.1–0.2 mg/kg i/m when in CHF, otherwise 0.3–0.5 mg/kg q4–6h
	Cat	0.1 mg/kg q6–8h
Pimobendan	Dog	0.1–0.3 mg/kg q12h po on an empty stomach

DRUG GLOSSARY

DRUG GLOSSARY TABLE   (continued)

Drug	Species	Dose
Prednisolone	Dog/cat	1–2 mg/kg q12h po, reducing to 0.2 mg/kg q48h
Procainamide	Dog	2 mg/kg i/v bolus, repeat to response, up to a maximum of 15 mg/kg in 20 min
Propantheline	Dog	0.5–2 mg/kg q8h po
Bromide	Cat	7.5 mg q8–12h
Propranolol	Dog	0.2–2 mg/kg q8h po (start at lowest dose)
	Cat	2.5 mg q8h po, up to 5 mg q8h
	Dog/cat	0.01–0.1 mg/kg i/v (start low and titrate up)
Ramipril	Dog	0.125 mg/kg q24h po (increase to q12h in advanced cases)
Rutin	Dog/cat	50 mg/kg q8h
Sodium Nitroprusside	Dog	1.0–5.0 µg/kg/min i/v
Sotalol	Dog	0.5–2 mg/kg q12h po
Spironolactone	Dog	Diuretic dose: 1–4 mg/kg q12–24h.
	Cat	Diuretic dose: 1–2 mg/kg q12–24h
		Note: Anti-aldosterone dose is probably $1/4$ of the diuretic dose.
Streptokinase	Cat	90 000 iu over 30 min, then 45 000 iu/h for 3–6 h
Taurine	Dog	500 mg q12h
	Cat	250 mg q12h
Terbutaline	Dog	1.25–5 mg per dog q8–12h po
	Cat	0.625–1.25 mg per cat q8–12h po
Theophylline	Dog	10–20 mg/kg q12h po
	Cat	20 mg/kg q12–24h
Verapamil	Dog	0.05 mg/kg i/v every five minutes to effect (to a maximum of 0.15 mg/kg in 10–15 min)
	Cat	0.025 mg/kg i/v

REFERENCES

Bayon, A., Fernandez Del Palacio, M.J., Montes, A.M., *et al.* (1994) M-mode echocardiographic study in growing Spanish mastiffs. *Journal of Small Animal Practice*, 35:473–9.

Bonagura, J.D., O'Grady, M.R. & Herring, D.S. (1985) Echocardiography: Principles of interpretation. *Veterinary Clinics of North America: Small Animal Practice*, 15:1177–94.

Boon, J. (1998) *Manual of Veterinary Echocardiography*. Williams & Wilkins, Pennsylvania.

Brownlie, S.E. & Cobb, M.A. (1999) Observations on the development of congestive heart failure in Irish wolfhounds with dilated cardiomyopathy. *Journal of Small Animal Practice*, 40:371–7.

Brownlie, S.E. (1999) A cardiac auscultation, electrocardiographic and echocardiographic study in Salukis. *Clinical Research Abstract*, BSAVA Congress, p. 243.

Crippa, L., Ferro, E., Melloni, E., *et al.* (1992) Echocardiographic parameters and indices in the normal Beagle dog. *Lab Animals*, 26:190–5.

Day, M.J. & Martin, M.W.S. (2002) Immunohistochemical characterisation of the lesions of canine idiopathic pericarditis. *Journal of Small Animal Practice*, 43:382–7.

Dukes-McEwan, J. (1999) Echocardiographic/Doppler criteria of normality: The findings in cardiac disease and the genetics of familial dilated cardiomyopathy in Newfoundland dogs. PhD thesis, University of Edinburgh.

Gooding, J.P., Robinson, W.F. & Mews, G.C. (1986) Echocardiographic assessment of left ventricular dimensions in clinically normal English Cocker Spaniels. *American Journal of Veterinary Research*, 47:296–300.

Häggström, J., Hansson, K., Kvart, C., *et al.* (2000) Secretion patterns of the natriuretic peptides in naturally acquired mitral regurgitation attributable to chronic valvular disease in dogs. *Journal of Veterinary Cardiology*, 2:7–16.

Herrtage, M. (1994) Echocardiographic measurements in the normal Boxer. *Proceedings of the 4th ESVIM* 172–4.

Jacobs, G. & Knight, D.H. (1985) M-mode echocardiographic measurements in nonanaesthetized healthy cats: Effects of body weight, heart rate, and other variables. *American Journal of Veterinary Research*, 46:1705.

Koch, J., Pedersen, H.D., Jensen, A.L. & Flagstad, A. (1996) M-mode echocardiographic diagnosis of dilated cardiomyopathy in giant breed dogs. *Journal of the Veterinary Medical Association*, 43:297–304.

Macintire, D.K. (1995) The practical use of constant-rate infusions. In: *Kirk's Current Veterinary Therapy XII* (ed J.D. Bonagura), pp. 184–8. WB Saunders, Philadelphia.

Martin, M. (2000) *Small Animal ECGs: An Introductory Guide*. Blackwell Science, Oxford.

Morrison, S.A., Moise, N.S., Scarlett, J., *et al.* (1992) Effect of breed and body weight on echocardiographic values in four breeds of dogs of differing somatotype. *Journal of Veterinary Internal Medicine*, 6:220–4.

O'Grady, M.R. & Horne, R. (1995) Echocardiographic findings in 51 normal Dobermann pinschers. ACVIM abstract in: *Journal of Veterinary Internal Medicine*, 9:202.

Page, A., Edmunds, G. & Atwell, R.B. (1993) Echocardiographic values in the greyhound. *Australian Veterinary Journal*, 70:361–3.

Rishniw, M. & Erb, H.N. (2000) Evaluation of four 2-dimensional echocardiographic methods of assessing left atrial size in dogs. *Journal of Veterinary Internal Medicine*, 14:429–35.

Sisson, D. & Schaeffer, D. (1991) Changes in linear dimensions of the heart, relative to body weight as measured by M-mode echocardiography in growing dogs. *American Journal of Veterinary Research*, 52:1591–6.

Stafford Johnson, M., Martin, M., Binns, S. & Day, M.J. (2004) A retrospective study of clinical findings, treatment and outcome in 143 dogs with pericardial effusion. *Journal of Small Animal Practice*, 45:546–52.

Tilley, L.P. (1992) *Essentials of Canine and Feline Electrocardiography*, 3rd edn. Lea & Febiger, Philadelphia.

Vollmar, A.C. (1998) Kardiologische Untersuchungen beim Deerhound, Referenzwerte fur die Echodiagnostik. *Kleintierpraxis*, 43:497–508.

Vollmar, A.C. (1999a) Echocardiographic measurements in the Irish wolfhound: Reference values for the breed. *Journal of the American Animal Hospitals Association*, 35:271–7.

Vollmar, A.C. (1999b) Use of echocardiography in the diagnosis of dilated cardiomyopathy in Irish wolfhounds. *Journal of the American Animal Hospitals Association*, 35:279–83.

REFERENCES

INDEX

Note: page numbers in *italics* refer to tables.

INDEX

Summary of the procedures in cardiopulmonary resuscitation (Dr ABC)

	Procedure	Comments
D – Danger	**Assess situation**	Beware of bite/scratch wounds to personnel
R – Response	**Check response**	Assess level of consciousness
A – Airway	**Establish an airway – intubate**	Check airway is not occluded
B – Breathing	**Positive pressure ventilation** at 25–30/min with 100% oxygen	Ensure there is a supranormal chest-wall excursion and allow lungs to deflate fully
C – Circulation		
Small Dog or Cat	By the **cardiac pump mechanism** • Compression rate = 80–120/min • Ventilate during each second or third compression	Small, narrow-chested animals, cats and puppies with good chest-wall compliance, weighing <20 kg
Large Dog	By the **thoracic pump mechanism** • *Plus* abdominal binding	Broad-chested and large animals weighing >20 kg
Poor Response *Large Dog*	Consider **internal cardiac massage** • *Plus* cross clamping of the descending aorta	Broad-chested and large animals weighing >20 kg Any animal with a poor response to external cardiac compression
D – Drugs	**Asystole** • Atropine • Methoxamine • Adrenaline **Electromechanical dissociation** • Dexamethasone • Methoxamine • Calcium • Adrenaline • Bicarbonate **Sinus bradycardia** • Atropine • Beta agonist, e.g. dobutamine or dopamine	Minimise hypothermia Fluid loading Minimise hypothermia
E – Electrical Defibrillation	**Idioventricular rhythm** **Ventricular fibrillation** • Requires electrical defibrillation • Remember to maintain CPR between shocks	Poor prognosis Unlikely to be successful without electrical defibrillation Try precordial thump
F – Follow-up	• Fluids • Dopamine or dobutamine may be required • High dose of steroids and hyperventilation • Catheterise bladder and monitor rate of urine production • Irrigate chest to clean and warm • Close thoracotomy and ensure analgesia with nerve block • Maintain PPV until spontaneous breathing is established • Supply oxygen by nasal catheter during recovery	